The Dauntless
Nurse

Communication Confidence Builder

MARTHA GRIFFIN, RN, PHD

KATHLEEN BARTHOLOMEW, RN, MN

ARNA ROBINS, RN, MSN

The Dauntless Nurse: Communication Confidence Builder is published by Martha E. Griffin, Kathleen Bartholomew, and Arna Robins.

ISBN: 978-1-537-27724-0

Advice given is general. Readers should consult professional counsel for specific legal, ethical, or clinical questions. Note that the names of the doctors and nurses in this book are fictitious.

Arrangements can be made for quantity discounts. For more information, contact kathleenbart@msn.com.

Preface

Carol is a 38-year-old, well-educated, accomplished nurse with a Bachelor's degree and 15 years' work experience in the burn trauma intensive care unit. She has a reputation for doing a good job with direct patient care, but is feared by many of her colleagues. No one ever wants to give or take report from her. Carol routinely comes in 45 minutes before her shift and trolls the assignment sheet. If anyone questions her actions, she barks out, "I'm assessing the suck factor in my assignment, and making adjustments." She then waits until it is exactly start time and walks slowly toward her colleagues to receive report. The nurse manager has met with her many times about the aura she projects, but Carol repeatedly retorts, "Oh, that's just how we nurses are!"

If you've ever had a similar experience, this book is for you. These learned behaviors are not "how we nurses are." These behaviors start year one, semester one, and begin a pattern of negative, verbal, and non-verbal conduct that is repeated through mimicry, but can be "deleted" through education.

As authors, we've had these types of experiences too, and have been drawn together by our common desire to stop them.

Many years ago when Martha was a student, she was in the bookstore and had just picked up a large text for a class when a women blurted out, "Are you in this class?!" Startled, she nervously answered, "Yes." That's when the lady retorted, "I wrote that book, and I teach that class. Most students have to take it twice before they pass." Then, she just walked away. To this day, Martha wonders why this instructor felt the need to be so intimidating.

The hundreds of stories we have listened to with sadness, dismay, and concern, have motivated us to write this book. Every single scenario in this book is real.

It is time to create a new story—the story of a profession where nurses care as deeply for each other as they do for their patients. Whether you are in school studying to become a nurse, or are already immersed in the clinical arena, our goal is to provide a practical field guide for navigating professional practice.

For the love of nursing, let's raise the bar!

— Martha, Kathleen and Arna

We've all chosen to do this with our lives.
So it better be damn good. It better be worth it.

— Steve Jobs

About the Authors

Martha E. Griffin, RN, CS, PH.D., FAAN

An accomplished nurse leader, educator and researcher, Martha E. Griffin speaks nationally on raising the level of professionalism in nursing practice and improving women's access to healthcare insurance. Dr. Griffin has been long recognized for her positive influence on nursing and patient safety as a result of her research and writing on the subject of lateral violence. Her important work includes techniques to identify the most frequent forms of lateral violence and recognize their effect on nurses, as well as interventions to use when issues arise. Her 2004 and 2014 publications generated insight and interest throughout the nursing community, particularly as the research related to the impact of these behaviors on the most vulnerable population of nurses—nursing students and nurses new to practice.

Kathleen Bartholomew, RN, MN

Kathleen Bartholomew, internationally renowned speaker and educator, uses the power of story and her strong background in sociology to illuminate and trans-form the healthcare culture. The author of *Speak Your Truth: Proven Strategies for Effective RN-MD Communication*, and the bestseller *Ending Nurse-to-Nurse Hostility*, she is also co-author of *Charting the Course*. For over 15 years, Kathleen has inspired countless audiences of medical professionals to embrace an entirely new model of cooperative practice based on collegiality and honest communication. She has worked tirelessly from the bedside to the boardroom to raise awareness about patient safety, leadership, and culture, inspiring nurses to pursue both the art and science of nursing.

https://www.youtube.com/watch?v=Qh4HW3yx00w

Arna Robins, RN, MSN, CEN, CFRN, NREMT

Arna Robins obtained her BSN from Azusa Pacific University and her MSN from Grand Canyon University. A flight nurse for over a decade, she specialized in transporting critically ill neonatal and pediatric patients. While working on her Master's capstone project she became an advocate for ending lateral violence in nursing through developing and rehearsing communication skills. Her project focus wove communication exercises and role-play through every semester of undergraduate nursing. Her writing can be found in *The Examined Life Journal* and at Azusa Pacific University. She highly recommends all medical personnel view one ZDoggMD episode a day to maintain humor and outside-the-box thinking.

Table of Contents

How Dauntless Are You?

- Pre-test your communication skills by taking the test on page 83. Starting score: _____

- Re-take the test after reading the book and note your new score here: _____

Introduction

Nurses must be as proficient in communication skills as they are in clinical skills.

—AACN Standards for Nursing

Assertive communication is the single most vital skill you can possess as a nurse in the 21st century. Without assertive communication skills, nurses doubt themselves, make mistakes, and put themselves and their patients in danger. Why? Because in a psychologically unsafe and emotionally unsupportive environment, humans cannot think straight, let alone access the critical thinking skills that are essential to provide quality nursing care.

The tools and tips in this handbook will give you the knowledge and skills you need to confidently address experiences and behaviors that leave you feeling undermined or uncertain. Understanding why these behaviors occur lessens their effect. Knowing how to respond will build your confidence and hardwire muscle memory. And reading scenarios of how other nurses have effectively handled similar situations will empower you to be dauntless.

Dauntless?

You may ask, what is so important about the word dauntless that we chose it for the title of this handbook? And why is the term important for nurses?

---

dauntless [dawnt-lis, dahnt-les]
Synonyms: brave, intrepid, valiant, audacious, courageous
adjective **1.** not to be daunted or intimidated; fearless; intrepid; bold: a dauntless hero.
The history of the world is peopled with dauntless men and women who refused to be subdued or "tamed" by fear.

In the 1850's, Florence Nightingale called for her students of nursing to be just that—dauntless—because she recognized that they needed this trait to be successful professionals. The need today to be resolute, fearless, and bold is just as great—if not greater.

Because the keyboard is a useful tool used by nearly everyone to communicate, we've chosen to use the universal PC keyboard "reboot" key combination Control+Alt+Delete as our shorthand for rebooting challenging or difficult conversations.

Our minds run like computers. When your computer freezes, crashes or does weird things, you re-boot. This handbook will show you how and when to "Control+Alt+Delete" the disempowering conversations that have a dramatic and sustained effect on how you feel, and thus how you practice. (If you're not a PC user and don't use this bit of keyboard magic, don't worry. Just follow along. You won't be sorry.)

In this book, you'll also find other simple techniques to become a more fearless and proactive nurse and team member. We look at Construct/Deconstruct, which is another way to reset/reboot situations. We'll spend a fair amount of time identifying and categorizing different types of verbal and non-verbal lateral violence, so that you can recognize them when you experience them. And we'll give you specific scripts you can memorize and use when you find yourself in uncomfortable situations. We call this Cognitive Rehearsal, and in our final chapter, we share with you a set of twenty stories from real nurses who have used the techniques in this book to become more dauntless, just as you will.

But I will find new habits, new thoughts, new rules. I will become something else.

—Veronica Roth, *Divergent*

What You Can Expect

From beginning to end, this handbook provides you with indispensable communication tools that will have a powerful effect on your relationships at work and at home. Work through the chapters in this handbook and you'll take important steps to hardwire your communication "muscle memory." Here's how we do it, one chapter at a time:

Chapter 1: Facing the Challenge of Lateral Violence

Why You Gotta Be So Mean? You will see that negative behaviors are learned behaviors with a powerful pull because, as humans, we copy what we see others doing without questioning. In this chapter, you'll learn that when you control your inner dialogue, you have the power to create a new story and; therefore, a new response.

Chapter 2: Expecting the Best from Your Team

Am I Asking Too Much? Chapter 2 invites us to stop and take a minute to look at our expectations. What do you do if what you expect is different from your everyday reality? It's not easy to question the way we've always done things, but it helps to know that only a cohesive team can keep our patients safe.

Chapter 3: Good (and Bad) Group Dynamics

Join the Club! This chapter helps us to understand group dynamics and why cliques exist. We examine what happens when you confront a group. We show you how to make the group's behaviors visible without stirring up the beehive.

Chapter 4: Identifying Negative Learned Behaviors

Why Does It Feel So Normal? Here you'll learn how to stay in your truth and power. You will become mindful of your good guesses and will learn how to take them apart. You can change any situation by your response, but you can't change your external world until you change your internal dialogue.

Chapter 5: Shades of (Unacceptable) Behavior

Call It What It Is! Chapter 5 describes the most common forms of lateral violence: favoritism, cliques, ignoring, rudeness, and intimidation, eye-rolling, blaming, and backstabbing, just to name a few. We give you a specific example of each so you can call them what they are!

Chapter 6: Choosing Your Role in a Hostile Work Environment

Ouch! This chapter helps take the sting out of lateral violence. You'll learn that everyone is dramatically impacted by these hurtful behaviors. We look at the role of the victim, bully, and witness, and teach you the D-E-S-C communication tool.

Chapter 7: Preparing Yourself with Cognitive Rehearsal

What Do I Do Again? Here we offer you yet another tool—Cognitive Rehearsal. You learn specifically how to respond to scapegoating, rudeness, rolling eyes, cliques, and favoritism. When you say what you see and validate the facts, you can communicate your way to great professional relationships.

Chapter 8: Dauntless Trailblazers

Building Resilience and Becoming Fearless. In this chapter you'll learn from the experiences of other nurses and nurse leaders who have incorporated the use of D-E-S-C, Ctrl+Alt+Delete, and Cognitive Rehearsal into their day-to-day conversations. Remember: *Power=Voice.*

Afterword: Self-Reflection

Am I a Bully? Are any of the behaviors described in the book a bit too familiar? Our final words encourage you to reflect on your own behaviors.

The book ends with two appendices—one that you can use to test what you've learned and another with resources and the research referenced in the book.

CHAPTER 1

Facing the Challenge of Lateral Violence
Why You Gotta Be So Mean?

Not knowing why negative behaviors are happening is debilitating and weakens our sense of self-esteem. Knowing why

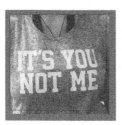

these behaviors are happening and how they started is the first step to stopping them.

In order to stand in your own power, you need to know unequivocally, as the Victoria's Secret t-shirt says:

> *It's you, not me.*

Understanding Lateral Violence

A large percentage of nursing professionals refuse to even discuss the possibility that lateral violence exists within the profession, fearing that to do so would denigrate the profession (Mitchell, Ahmed, & Szabo, 2014). Still others believe that not talking about lateral violence somehow prevents the behavior from existing or growing in their organization.

The reality, however, is that success and cohesion within our profession will only come from appreciative inquiry; from understanding why lateral violence exists, and by individual actions which then make lateral violence obsolete.

The Imbalance of Power

For the past two decades, nurses have explored theories and models of oppressed group behavior to explain their subordinated, powerless position as a group of mostly women in a male-dominated society. Nurse-on-nurse relational aggression (or why nurses eat their young) is best understood as oppressed group behaviors (OGB).

In *Pedagogy of the Oppressed* (1971), Paulo Friere asked:

> *What happens in groups of people when some people have (or perceive) more power than others?*

After observing numerous groups of people, Friere concluded that when a dominant group exerts power on an oppressed group, the oppressed group cannot direct its power upward. Because the oppressed group needs an outlet for their frustration, they unconsciously direct their anger/energy toward each other by infighting. They forget what they value and start measuring them- selves by the dominant group values, so their self-esteem drops and a cycle of oppression reboots in our everyday interactions.

The Roots of Oppression in Nursing

The evolution of nursing provides another clue. Reflecting on the role of women in the late 1800's into the early 1900's gives us insight into when and how both positive and negative aspects of nursing culture developed. The nursing profession's historical link to the Army, and the influence of the military on nursing, particularly related to the Nightingale Schools of Nursing, is well documented (Hadikin & O'Driscoll, 2000).

The early curricula for *Nursing and Midwifery Education* listed "boldness" and "dauntlessness" as subjects to be taught. It is theorized that these behavioral characteristics were needed to care for strangers because nursing was a new profession that broke the societal norms for women. Emphasizing these characteristics in nursing practice served to override Victorian era expectations for women's behavior.

The framework for virtually all contemporary nursing educational programs derives from the early formation of the Nightingale schools, an approach that has carried on throughout the generations. Consider this, more contemporary, example:

One day I was talking with my aunt who is a nurse and she said, "I was in the 50% of the class that graduated, so that's all that mattered."

"What do you mean 50%? Did half the class actually fail?" I asked.

"Yes," she replied matter-of-factly. "The instructors were told to weed out the weak ones. One day I was making a bed and my instructor came around the corner, and in a loud, harsh voice shouted, 'What are you doing?!' I remained calm and did not flinch. I replied, 'I am making a bed.' You see, she was just trying to toughen us up for the doctors, and I passed her test."

Inherited Codes of Nursing Behavior

DNA is not the only thing that is passed down through generations. *Memes* are the names given to cultural codes of behavior that are passed on through- out many generations (Francisco Gil-White, 2001).

The cultural meme for nursing instructors was to be tough because they understood that women in a very patriarchal society (especially in a new profession working with people who were vulnerable, naked, and frightened) needed to be extremely strong (Dauntless!). However, nursing faculty could not separate the role of woman and nurse, so these prevalent beliefs dominated:

- *Women are property*
- *Silence is golden—don't speak until spoken to*

7

- *Nurses must serve physicians dutifully and without fault*

- *Women are inferior to men*

- *Don't rock the boat*

Intimidation Tactics

In the Victorian era, nurses mopped and dusted, trimmed wicks, cleaned chimneys, cared for fifty patients, worked seven days a week with one evening off for courting, etc. As a result of these demanding expectations, our cultural memes were established. Instructors learned behavioral tactics designed to intimidate—a practice that persists today as they (and we) copy the behaviors of our predecessors. Here is an example of intimidating behavior you may encounter:

> *An orthopedic operating room nurse is asked to fill in for a cardiac nurse who is on vacation. As soon as she enters the operating room, the cardiac surgeon looks up and makes a disappointed face and then refuses to make eye contact at all during the operation.*

Students have consequently acquired the messages embedded in the instructors' behaviors and incorporated them into their own conduct, as shown in the following student's anecdote:

> *My problem is more with fellow classmates. If I ask a question in class that seems silly, they would clearly utter a judgmental tone or comment. And I've had situations where I did not know what to do and I was not given an explanation at all. Instead, I would get this sudden cold feeling in the air, if you know what I mean.*

As students become independent nurses themselves, they perpetuate the learned behaviors they observe in other professionals in the field and those learned in schools. They then inflict the same behaviors on other aspiring nurses:

Almost every clinical experience day when I walk up to the nurses' station looking for a nurse to partner with that day, I get the disgusted, eye-rolling looks in return.

The Arrival of the Millennial Nurse

It's difficult to view the perspective of women and the early development of professional nursing from the Millennial nurse's mind and timeframe because it was so very long ago. However, doing so adds insight into the evolution of the acculturated behaviors of our contemporary colleagues.

Remember, these are **learned behaviors**. The best hope for change is in a new generation of nurses who create their own set of new memes, where the underlying belief is different, based on a sense of balance, worthiness, and self-esteem.

New, Millennial nurses are savvy, quick, connected, and value a work-life balance. It's possible that we can learn from them and establish new standards and positive beliefs, like the following:

*I can be strong **and** professional at the same time. Nurses must support and nurture each other at all times.*

There is no place for fear and intimidation in such a noble profession. Only by functioning as a collegial team can we keep our patients safe.

The only hope for changing learned behaviors is to understand how and why these behaviors originate, and to then ask how do we make them go away? The answer is simple—fortified with a new set of beliefs and principles—we use our knowledge to construct a new reality. In short, we create a new reality for ourselves and our profession!

TOOL: Control+Alt+Delete

Reinterpreting Uncomfortable Situations

Just like on a computer keyboard, reboot your thinking using **Control+Alt+Delete**. (Note: Mac users will have to trust us that on PCs this magic combination is the key to getting out of all manner of sticky situations.)

Here's how you can use the Control+Alt+Delete tool to "show up" and respond to difficult situations:

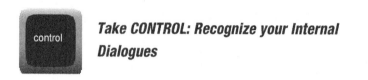

Take CONTROL: Recognize your Internal Dialogues

1. The first thing you need to do is recognize your internal landscape. What are you thinking? What's your self-talk? Your internal dialogue must change first in order for the external dialogue to be meaningful and productive. Are you thinking:

   The nurse rolled her eyes so she must not want to work with me today.

   If this is your self-talk, you're likely to interpret and act negatively:

   - **What you think**: Is there something wrong with me? Or being a student? Or this profession? What did I get myself into?

   - **What you decide**: I'm going to lay low.

Use ALT: Reframe your Interpretation

2. **Your new interpretation:** When you look for an alternative reason for the eye-rolling behavior (one that acknowledges external factors), you may develop a less personal interpretation:

I noticed the nurse rolled her eyes when she realized that she was with a student today.

With a reframed assessment, you realize that it isn't all about you. You can develop a more self-assured self-talk:

I've learned that because of a perceived lack of power, mostly based on gender, nurses developed a culture of infighting that has nothing to do with me, but everything to do with my feeling capable and confident in my new role.

Press DELETE: Create a New Response

3. With this new perspective on your uncomfortable situation, you can create the kind of response that would make any dauntless nurse proud:

I need to speak with her now.

Now You Know

- It's not about you, so don't take it personally.

- These negative behaviors are learned behaviors. (We copy what we see.)

- You control your inner dialogue.

- New thoughts = new responses.

- This is how a new cultural meme is born. (One response at a time—yours!)

You, with your words like knives and swords and weapons that you use against me. You have knocked me off my feet again got me feeling like I'm nothing. You, with your voice like nails on a chalk- board, calling me out when I'm wounded...all you're ever gonna be is mean.

—Taylor Swift
www.youtube.com/watch?v=jYaleI1hpDE

CHAPTER 2

Expecting the Best from Your Team
Am I Asking Too Much?

Our sense of self is not something that we solely control: furthermore, it is not something that can be divorced from how we see and are seen by others.

-J.R. Clippinger, 2007

You have the right to be treated with respect and professional courtesy at all times. Research shows that the self-esteem of nurses is parallel to that of graduates of other departments such as biology or business, but for nurses this self-esteem falls after graduation. The process of assimilation into the nursing culture often deflates our sense of self-worth.

This progression begins primarily because of the overt, non-verbal gestures such as eye-rolling, ignoring, and raised eyebrows that are common in the nursing profession and among women in general (Simmons, 2011). Left unexplained, these ambiguous non-verbal behaviors increase stress and decrease self-esteem.

Ambiguity is like walking on thin ice because you never know when or if you are going to fall through. For example, did the charge nurse give you the most difficult and time-consuming patient on the floor on purpose, or did she not realize the patient's complexity?

Without clear communications, your expectations about respect and your ability to provide safe nursing care are at risk.

The Impact of Non-Verbal Cues

In fact, the most impactful way that humans communicate is not with their words—**non-verbal cues** affect us the most. Examples of this:

A lead instructor of mine rolls her eyes and huffs when asked a question. This makes not only the person asking the question uncomfortable, but others that may have questions refuse to approach her.

I needed to give an RN an update on a patient's status. She didn't have time to discuss it with me. To her, students are an encumbrance. As she was walking down the hall she said, "Come on, just follow me and tell me what you wanted to ask me." I told her that I didn't have a question, although our patient had no pedal pulses.

What was the impact of this instructor's non-verbal cues? The student was too intimidated to share her knowledge of the patient's health, and too fearful to ask a question critical to the patient's safety.

The student had the right attitude—using the term "our" patient. When you're on the unit you may hear the possessive adjective "my" used more frequently, but don't buy into this culture. The only way we can keep patients safe is if we form a team for our patients every day, and ask important questions when they arise, because questions are the conduit to knowledge, and **knowledge is what keeps patients safe**.

Preventable Hospital Errors

The one thing you can count on as a new nurse is that you'll make a mistake. We all make mistakes because we're humans working in time-compressed, high risk, stressful environments.

There is always a second victim when a patient suffers as the result of a mistake—the healthcare professional who made the mistake experiences guilt and trauma as well. Sometimes the cost is a human life, permanent damage (both visible and invisible), or a revoked license. Unfortunately, these events occur more frequently than previously thought. The following illustrates a real-life example:

> We recognized the signs and symptoms of a stroke and transferred the micro-discectomy patient to the ICU after he started to have severe chest pain. The new nurse in the ICU—with less than a year's experience—did a great job managing his cardiac problems, but she forgot to check his pedal pulses. In the morning he was rushed to emergency surgery, but it was too late. Now this 52-year-old man is a paraplegic. Maybe if she felt safe asking, "Is there anything I've forgotten?" to her peers, his story would have turned out differently.

It is the responsibility and duty of every nurse to create an environment where peers aren't afraid to speak up because they might be perceived as stupid or wrong or incompetent. How can you help create this atmosphere?

Speak Your Truth

The answer to the previous question sounds deceptively simple: **Always speak your truth and say what is on your mind.** But what if no one listens?

> I couldn't hear breath sounds and no one would listen to check. Eventually another nurse backed me up and an x-ray was ordered. The patient had full white-out lung, septic shock, and pneumothorax. It wasn't until the patient's BP crashed that the PA felt the need to listen, but by then the doctor and I were palpating a pulse and trying

to stabilize. This patient spent 14 days in the ICU under sedation, on a ventilator.

The IOM report of 1999 found that up to 98,000 patients die a year from infections acquired in the hospital and accidents **that were preventable.** Then, in 2013, researchers found that this early estimate was grossly under- stated. More than 400,000 people die every year because of preventable mistakes and through acquired infections (James, 2012).

To put this number in perspective, 400,000 deaths is the equivalent of nearly 1,200 fully loaded Boeing 747's crashing every year, or three planes every day. Can you imagine the public outcry if even a small fraction of this number actually crashed each year? The result would be instantaneous and catastrophic for the airline industry. People would simply stop flying.

As it is, hospital errors are the third leading cause of death in the United States. Your baggage is safer on any airline than patients are in our hospitals. In fact, you are exponentially safer on any airline than you would be as a patient. Why?

Aviation radically changed its culture after the catastrophic crash of two Boeing 747s on March 24, 1977 at Tenerife—and the corresponding horrific visual effect of 583 body bags. When experts listened to the cockpit recordings they discovered that this disaster was most attributable to a hierarchical culture in the cockpit. The first mate was afraid to speak up to warn the captain of one of the planes that he didn't have permission for take-off.

Teamwork and High Reliability Institutions

High reliability industries realize that only a culture of collegiality and teamwork can keep people safe. These organizations created a new culture based on a set of principles and beliefs that have been demonstrated to maintain high quality in high risk situations.

By definition, a high reliability organization is an organization that manages an inherent risk with great precision and few, if any, serious accidents or incidents ever occur. The term was first coined by Karl Weick (2015), who discovered consistently superior performance in particular organizations where there was a high potential for danger and error (like nuclear power plants or high rise skyscrapers). Weick coined the phrase "highly reliable" because the errors they experienced were caught and corrected **before** they progressed to a catastrophe.

Team Work Is Critical to Patient Safety

The negative effect that bullying behaviors have on the safety of our patients and on our profession in general cannot be minimized.

I was in my first week cross-training into the special procedures unit. We were preparing to receive a patient, and my preceptor told me we needed a different tray with specialized instruments. She told me to stay in the room and set up what was already there and she would go find the tray. Minutes later, the team arrived with the patient.

One of the nurses noticed the requested tray was absent, and commented on that. Before I could explain that my preceptor had gone to retrieve it, she came back into the room and said to me, "It was right where I said it was." Then, she looked at the nurse who had made the comment and said, "She's new—you know how it goes." I realized at that moment I was on my own.

If healthcare functioned as a highly reliable organization, our patients would be safe and we would be protected by the system from causing harm. Part of this protection comes from creating a collegial interactive team (Nance, 2010). Therefore, working as a team is aligned with our ethical obligation to "First Do No Harm", as evidenced by the experience of a group of nurses:

> *During clinical rounds our group was placed on a unit that was severely understaffed. At first we were a bit daunted by how many high-acuity patients each nurse was assigned, but we soon rallied together and began working as a team to help the nurses on the unit. Not only did we learn a lot this day, the staff nurses were so grateful for our help and we all felt great about the day we each had.*

Good teams are respectful, encouraging, honest, and have open communication because they realize that **their relationships with each other are the safety net that will catch human error**. It's the patient that benefits the most when we work together, and the patient who is put in a vulnerable and potentially dangerous position when we are pitted against one another.

One of the most critical aspects is that the best teams are **non-hierarchical**—no one person thinks they are better than, worth more, or more important than another. While there are many great teams in healthcare, we have a long way to go as evidenced by new nurses still experiencing the hierarchy in both overt and covert ways. For example, you'll see nurses picking up the phone and beginning a call to the physician with an apology, or a physician assistant acting superior to a nurse who then, in turn, is bossy to a nursing assistant.

Question: How do I know if I have experienced horizontal hostility?

Answer: You feel "less than" another person after an interaction.

Defining Critical Expectations

How do you expect to be treated as a new nurse? Stop for a full minute and write down the answer to this question.

_____

_____

_____

Your expectations are critical because they form the framework for how you perceive and make sense of the way that people act around you. They decide whether you'll say something, or stay silent.

Your expectations are like a set of eye glasses. Through these expectation lenses we decide if things are going well or if they are not; if the problem is me or them. We use the answers to these questions to form an opinion of ourselves (I am a good nurse; or I am a failure).

How Are You Being Treated?

We derive a sense of **self** through our interactions with others (Clippinger, 2007). Social emotions are critical because they form our identity.

Take a minute to write down how you are being treated as a new-to-practice nurse, or a new nurse to a unit, or even an experienced nurse. Does your treatment match your expectations?

_____

_____

_____

_____

Your challenge is to close the gap between how you expect to be treated and how you are treated. In order for you to be a sane,

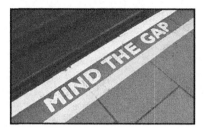

successful, and competent team player, you must be treated as you expect to be treated. As they say in Europe, *"Mind the gap!"*

The New Nursing Memes

Hospitals today have embraced the principles of high reliability organizations and teamwork, and a new set of memes is growing in the nursing profession, as evidenced by the following recent experiences of student nurses. These are examples of how you should expect to be treated:

From the Instructor

When I removed stitches for the first time, the clinical instructor looked at the patient and said, "You're in good hands. She is very good."

To my surprise, upon initial assessment the patient had pulled out his NG tube and his blood sugar bottomed out. So here I am pushing D-50 and placing a new NG tube all in one day. In post conference my instructor told me, "You never flinched. You're a natural!"

I was starting an IV on a patient and felt that I found a good vein. My instructor didn't feel that it was a good vein and said as much. However, she also said that if I felt confident enough to go ahead and try. I started the IV in the vein I had chosen on the very first try and my instructor had nothing but praise for a job well done! She told me to always remain as confident with my skills as I was that day!

Each time my wonderful clinical instructor says to me, "Of course you can! I have confidence in you!" it makes me feel like I can conquer the world!

From New Nurses

I worked with a very skilled and very busy nurse. She gave me clear responsibilities and expectations and praised me when I met them. Once she was preoccupied with getting a patient onto a Hoyer lift and forgot to get the stretcher. I realized her mistake and asked her where she was going to move the patient to after he was lifted. She told me that I had been very observant and averted a potentially disastrous situation. I felt empowered by her frank praise and recognition of my value.

From Physicians

I was watching a bronchoscopy and was in the room with the team before the procedure started. The patient had a look of panic on his face while everyone moved around him hurriedly. I walked over and took his hand in mine. He blinked, looked up at me and smiled and said, "Thanks for saving an old man's heart." I told him he was in excellent hands. The room stopped and the doctor paused for a minute with a questioning look on his face. Before the doctor started the procedure he looked at me directly in the face and told me I certainly picked the right profession and he was more than proud to have me in the room. Talk about cloud nine!

Now You Know

- Your expectations determine what behaviors you'll respond to, tolerate, or ignore.

- Nursing is teamwork. Only teams keep patients safe.

- Our relationships are the safety net that catches error.

- Communication errors have the potential to translate to patient care errors.

CHAPTER 3

Good (and Bad) Group Dynamics

Join the Club!

> *The greatest need of the soul is for belonging.*
>
> —Thomas Moore

Human beings are neurologically hardwired to live in groups. Our primal selves are acutely aware of the fact that we cannot survive alone. Groups are so critical to our health and our psyche that just joining a group that meets once a month doubles our level of happiness, and cuts in half our odds of dying in the next year (www.BowlingAlone.com). We need each other.

Why Is the Group So Important to Nurses?

Belonging to the group is important to nurses because that is where you learn and develop nursing skills and knowledge. If the group isn't a safe place, we stop asking questions. If the group won't let us in, we feel alienated and withdraw into ourselves, feeling inadequate and alone.

There is not one new nurse who hasn't learned the tacit parts of nursing practice from anyone but another nurse. You may have heard experienced nurses saying that their nursing education began when "they hit the floor." What they are referring to is the vast body of knowledge that they learned from other nurses by observing and experiencing active repetitive patterns that were then validated.

In clinical situations, nurses learn by matching patterns. For students, there is a default to a procedure-driven process, book, or institutional materials like policy and procedures. But the ebb and flow of practice is actually learned while working with experienced nurses.

Another reason why the group is so important is because these nurses are the members of your team. No individual can ever be perfect all the time. We need a team of nurses who have our backs at all times; who are there to give us a helping hand or answer questions or notice that we have a lot on our minds at a particular time. All research clearly shows that our relationships with our peers form the safety net that will catch errors.

Hey, I'm New to the Group. What's Next?

The rest of the group teaches new members the group rules by using overt and covert behaviors. Think about the day of your first clinical experience—how long did it take you to learn who you could ask questions, and who you would never bother again? This process is called assimilation and it happens whenever one person joins an existing group.

Whenever people join a group, they quickly learn or try to learn the unspoken rules of what is "right" for that particular group.

Shelley had just finished her orientation and was working independently in the operating room one day when the surgeon requested an unfamiliar instrument and she hesitated. Suddenly the surgeon shot the preceptor a glance, and the preceptor deftly slapped the right instrument into the surgeon's hands. The preceptor shot Shelley a glance, and at the same time the surgeon rolled his eyes.

All groups have rules of behavior that we don't learn in school or orientation. Without ever speaking, everyone in the group agrees to these rules. What you permit, you promote; or, in other words, the behaviors that are allowed to occur over a period of time become the norms that form a particular culture. Anyone whose behavior, attitude, or language does not match the group, and/or anyone who challenges the group in any way, then becomes a threat to the group.

In fact, anyone who is different in any way is a threat. You could be too old, young, foreign, new, unique, unusual, upbeat, optimistic, or knowledgeable. It doesn't matter because, in the end, we function like the social animals we are. Let's look at some of the rules of behavior (the norms) you may encounter when you join a group in the workplace.

Healthy Group Norms

Here are some healthy group norms to recognize:

- The charge nurse assigns the lightest patient load to the preceptor.

- The preceptor asks for feedback from the new nurse saying, *"What can I do differently tomorrow that could help you learn better?"*

- When a staff member begins to talk about another person who isn't there, no one supports or engages in the conversation.

- When nurses are caught up with their work, they immediately offer to assist the other members of their team.

- Nursing assistants don't hesitate to ask a nurse for assistance, and their observations are valued as important. You can tell they feel valued and respected.

- Assignments are assessed continuously for equity based on acuity and experience.

- Nurses routinely complement each other and make sure that they all get a break.

- No one hesitates to ask a question when they don't know something.

What are some positive, healthy norms of your group?

_____

_____

_____

_____

Unhealthy Group Norms

Here are some unhealthy group norms to recognize:

- Certain nurses always come in late or take longer breaks.

- The nurse manager has a favorite who seems to get the lighter assignments.

- Nurses who smoke always seem to get their breaks.

- No one questions the nurse bully who has all the informal power.

- Some operating room nurses are drinking lattes, while the rest of the operating room staff is totally overwhelmed.

- Some nurses are so toxic that even the manager does not confront them.

- The charge nurse consistently gives the more experienced nurses the most complicated patients and they burn out.

What are some unhealthy norms of your group?

_____

_____

_____

_____

Cliques and Realistic Expectations

We all hope for an open, reciprocal, transparent environment where everyone realizes that no one is perfect and that we all make mistakes. We expect that nursing care must be delivered by a team in order to deliver high quality care safely because unexpected events happen all the time.

However, please don't expect an immediate invitation into a group that has been working together for years. Be patient. Decide how long you think it will take for you to be accepted into the group—and then add 2-3 months.

> ### TIP
>
> Don't assume it's about you. Never internalize the rejection and make it personal. Be a curious observer. Begin sentences with "I noticed that...."
>
> *I noticed that the same people always take their meal breaks together.*
> *I noticed that the group disbands when a new person tries to enter the conversation.*
> *I noticed that the smokers seem to get more breaks than the non-smokers.*

How Do I Deal with Cliques?

People form groups to stay safe and to raise their sense of self-esteem. If you see cliques, then you know that people at some point in time needed to bond together for psychological, emotional, or social safety. The reason they formed a clique was because they got something out of belonging to the group that they couldn't get as an individual (e.g., they had a bad manager from a decade ago). Group norms don't change quickly.

Cliques are groups of people that are bonded by association and have been connected with each other for a long period of time. Cliques are cloaked in invisibility and amass what they think is power by staying together at all costs. In Great Britain they call these "mobs." This terminology more accurately connotes the negative, devastating impact that a mob has on outsiders.

I was a new nurse on the labor and delivery night shift for six months. One night, after a particularly bad shift, the charge nurse said, "Let's go out for breakfast!"

"Where are you going?" I asked, but no one answered until someone finally mumbled, "The usual place." I went into the nurses' lounge and as I was putting things back in my locker, a nurse who felt sorry for me opened the door and said quickly, "We're going to the Pancake House." through the barely open door.

So I just went home. It hurt. It really hurt. We lost a baby that night and I felt so alone.

Dealing with Exclusion from the Group

You experience rejection, isolation, or exclusion—what do you do?

Don't assimilate into the group and match their behaviors. In other words, don't want to belong so badly that you do whatever the mob does so that they will accept you. The goal is to enter the group and be accepted *without matching their negative behaviors.*

For example, if you join the group, then perhaps you would choose to be consciously inclusive with all new nurses in the future after your own experiences and create a different norm.

Example: Let's use the example of the L&D nurse from above.

1. Analyze the situation. Be a CSI Agent (Communication Scene Investigator).

They are going to breakfast and you want to go, but you have clearly received the message that you are not invited from their ambiguous responses.

2. Say what you feel, sense or see. For example:

- *I sense that you don't want me to come to breakfast, is that the case?*

- *How do I become part of this group?*

- *It's difficult not to feel excluded right now.*

- *I am feeling left out. Is that your intention?*

- *What can I do to fit in or be accepted?*

- *How long did it take you to be accepted into this group?*

Possible Outcomes

1. They say, *"Of course you can come!"* and they mean it. It was just an oversight.

2. They default to humor, saying *"Of course you can come!"* but they don't mean it. What do you do? These words are still an invitation, so **accept** because you put it out there. To withdraw at this point is to play the game.

3. They say "no" whether verbally with sarcasm or innuendo. How critical is it that you join them today? Can you wait? How critical is this?

- **Not critical:** This is a second rejection. By continuing you would make yourself more vulnerable so you could send a message of inclusion, *"Maybe next time?"*

- **Critical:** You say, *"This has been a difficult shift and I need the support of my team right now. I'd like to come with you."*

Now You Know

- These people don't know you. They will reject anybody. *They can't reject you as a person, because they don't know you.* This is all about the group's safety and group think.

- Begin with the words *"I noticed that...."*

- You will get a response. Even no response is a response.

- When you call out a situation, express how you feel, and/or ask for a solution, you make the group's norms visible.

- Let it ride and be patient. If the situation does not change, rethink where you are working because patient outcomes, quality, safety, and learning depend on you being a part of a team. When you are alone, so is the patient.

Because true belonging only happens when we present our authentic, imperfect selves to the world, our sense of belonging can never be greater than our level of self-acceptance.

—Brené Brown, *Daring Greatly*

CHAPTER 4

Identifying Negative Learned Behaviors
Why Does It Feel So Normal?

One's dignity may be assaulted, vandalized and cruelly mocked, but it can never be taken away unless it is surrendered.

—Michael J. Fox

Culture is like looking at life through a pair of glasses that filter our perceptions. Whenever we join a new group we're handed a pair of these glasses which we are expected to wear as part of our initiation. This insidious process is called assimilation. We don't notice it because it happens so slowly—one interaction at a time.

Recognizing Embedded Negative Behaviors

Fatima is a newly licensed nurse who's worked in the orthopedic unit for six months. Lately she's felt that the assignments have been unfair, but she doesn't want to say anything to give the impression that she's not a hard worker. The last time she tried to speak up she met a wall of silence when the charge nurse embarrassed her in front of the rest of the team by saying, "Are you saying this assignment is too difficult for you?"

But today's assignment sheet validates her perceived pattern of injustice. Today Fatima has five patients, three of which are total care! The other nurses on the floor each have only one total care patient in their group. When Fatima starts to speak, all the other nurses hurry away, leaving her feeling that things are grossly unfair.

In Fatima's case, she learned quickly that it wasn't worth being labeled as lazy or incompetent by speaking up for herself.

These cultural frames help us adjust to the group. They tell us what we have to do to belong and to be accepted. Eventually, we forget that we even have perception altering lenses on at all. At the outset, new members of a group are much more likely to recognize the reality of a situation than long-time members because the more time that passes, the thicker the lenses become.

Some units have healthy, professional cultures as evidenced by feedback from members of a high-functioning organization:

I have never felt belittled.

I felt empowered after learning how to change batteries in cardiac monitoring devices because I was then the "go to" person to get the job done.

I took the lead for the day with a great nurse and did focus assessments, wound care, and medication administration. Just taking the lead and being confident in my nursing skills felt great.

The first time I inserted an IV with my clinical instructor I was nervous—my first two attempts were horrible. Then she guided my every move with a calm voice which led to a glorious flashback!

Other units have developed an unhealthy culture as evidenced by the following feedback:

A nurse saw me fumbling to get my hand placement right prior to drawing blood from a central line. She laughed at me and took the items right out of my hand and did it herself.

I was shadowing a nurse and a secretary asked why she bothered to take students because she knew most nurses just refused to work with them. My nurse replied, "It's not like I like them. I just feel bad and I have to take them." I was standing right in front of both of them.

Why Are Some Units Great and Others a Disaster?

The norms (what's considered "normal" in a culture) are determined by all the members of a group. If a manager consistently ignores bad behavior, then people know they can get away with it. If a manager is never on the floor and people only act badly when she or he is not there, then people know when they can get away with their negative behavior. If peers ignore the behavior of their peers, the behaviors continue. Even if a manager works diligently to address bad behavior but is blocked by human resources, he or she eventually stops trying.

The Pull to Their Normal

You will notice that even different shifts have subcultures and rules and feel unalike from one another. Each group builds its own particular norms by its everyday interactions, behaviors, and words. Note these facts about the pull to the group norm:

- It is easier to fit in and accommodate to the current culture.

- It is much more difficult to behave in a way that is contrary, or different than the group.

How to Stay on Track

Here are some tips on how to stay on track in the face of an unhealthy work culture.

- Always be fueled by the desire to work in a healthy culture.

- Never take these historical behaviors personally, which means internalizing them and doubting yourself and your abilities.

- Be the change agent for the profession, the patient, and yourself by learning role playing and rehearsing how to act in undermining and ambiguous situations.

- Learn how to use **Control+Alt+Delete** or the **Construct/Deconstruct** technique that follows in every challenging situation you encounter.

Construct/Deconstruct

If you're currently a nursing student or are a recent graduate, you may be familiar with the Construct/Deconstruct technique. The technique was developed by one of this book's authors, Martha Griffin, as an antidote to the lateral violence experienced by new-to- practice nurses. (Read more about Martha's lateral violence study here: *http://drlc4.com/Articles/files/304.pdf.*)

The Construct/Deconstruct technique can be used as an alternative to **Control+Alt+Delete**. The purpose is similar and the end results are the same—a new perspective and appropriate, assertive steps to take.

First, let's look at the key terms and their definitions.

Construct: Basically, a good guess as to why something is happening.

Definition: A working hypothesis/concept which represents the phenomenon on which you are focused at a point in time. It can be a behavior, concept, experience or incident.

Deconstruct: To take your best guess apart and question if it is true. Like a CSI agent (a Communication Scene Investigator), don't assume. Take the time to look at a situation from all angles with your new expert knowledge.

Definition: To take apart or examine in order to reveal the basis or composition of negative behaviors, often with the intention of exposing biases, flaws, or inconsistencies.

Construction/Deconstruction at Work

Let's apply Construction/Deconstruction to one of our earlier examples of negative behavior and look at the likely emotions involved and how the situation can be constructively addressed and remedied. You will recall this example:

A nurse saw me fumbling to get my hand placement correct prior to drawing blood from a central line. She laughed at me right in front of the patient, took the items right out of my hand and did it herself.

Construct

You have an experience like the one above. Immediately after the experience, whether you're aware of it or not, you create a story line to explain the event to yourself. This story line is called a **construct,** because you build (or *construct*) it out of your perception of the event. Some of the constructs for the above event might be:

I'm never going to learn anything here.

I wonder if I did something wrong? What was it? I need to know... I feel incompetent and humiliated. I don't want to come here tomorrow.

It's understandable that your first reaction may be to feel any (or all) of the above, but if you can put those thoughts away and recognize your value, you can build a new story line. This part of the process is critical to taking control of your perception (**Control**). Most of all, try not to personalize the event (it is never all about you), and then take these two key steps:

1. Take a deep breath and compose yourself.

2. Remember that the patient comes first, so wait until the task is completed before you respond.

Deconstruct

Dissect the event to better understand why, or how, it happened and if there was an opportunity in the moment for it to go differently. In this way you develop alternative (**Alt**) interpretations. Why do you need to deconstruct?

- The other nurse may have seen something your inexperienced eyes did not.

- The other nurse might have missed the teaching moment due to his or her own inexperience, distraction, or ignorance.

- The other nurse might just be mean, or simply venting frustration about other things going on in his or her life on you.

Applying the Deconstruction

The next steps are to form a new behavior based on your new, alternative interpretation. You reject the old story line (**Delete**) and create the new, more positive one.

3. In our example, your next move would be to ask to speak to the nurse in private, and be assertive.

   I need to speak to you in private now. The coffee room is free (or room 327 is empty, etc.).

4. You begin the conversation by describing *the* event and its impact on you, then pausing. Here are two possible conversation openers:

   When you laughed at me and took the supplies I felt humiliated.

   I don't understand your actions. In my experience, this was a teaching moment.

5. Finally, state what you want or need. For example:

6. *I needed your skill and knowledge, and I didn't get it. Can you guide me as to how you would do the procedure next time? I can see you are an expert, and I want to learn from you.*

Consider these possible responses:

- The skilled and experienced nurse saw something (air in the line, for example, or another potentially dangerous situation) and needed to intervene to prevent harm. She shares this with you.

- The other nurse says nothing. Silence is power and is blocking you out. Repeat yourself with the desire to "get on the same page."

- The other nurse walks away or leaves. In this case say, *"I would rather deal with this personally than going to my instructor. Will you stay and talk with me about it until we both feel alright?"*

- The nurse apologizes. You say, *"Thank you. I really look forward to learning from you, and I'm sorry that we got off to a rocky start for both of us."*

Can One Person Really Make a Difference?

Yes. One by one, as new members are assimilated into the group, the group norms slowly change. The nature of this transformation depends on your responses: whether you embrace, support and nurture others, ignore negative situations, or join the current culture by mimicking the behaviors you witness. This is where every single voice and action makes a difference.

Every interaction is critical (and the easiest way to be heard is to be prophylactic by complimenting a coworker every day).

The process of assimilating into a culture creates the veil. Every time you accommodate and say nothing to bad behavior, you are creating your own veil. Every time you ignore what you know is your truth, you betray yourself.

Using What You've Just Learned

Pretend you are Fatima in the opening story. How can you deconstruct this scene so that you are empowered **and** accepted by the group?

> *Today's assignment sheet validates Fatima's perceived pattern of injustice. Fatima has five patients and three of them are total care! All the other nurses on the floor only have one total care patient in their group. When she starts to speak, all the other nurses hurry away, leaving her feeling that things are grossly unfair.*

What Do You Do?

Ask to speak with the charge nurse in private, and say:

> *I wanted to make sure that you were aware that three of my five patients are total care. Even though I believe I am adjusting well to the unit, I don't believe that I, nor anyone else, can provide the type of care our patients deserve with this assignment. However, two total care patients would be manageable. Will you make an adjustment to the schedule?*

Now You Know

- Your conversation needs to happen as close to when the event occurred as possible.
- Soft eye contact with the desire to connect is more powerful than you can ever imagine. By soft eye contact, we mean that your eyes always say what you feel, so be gentle. Soft eye contact tells the other person that you are safe, and that they are safe because you aren't judging.
- Always hold the conversation in a private place.
- Begin assertively and be the broken record. If your request is denied or ignored, say it again until the person agrees to meet with you. Remember that the more they ignore you, the more frightened they are of the conversation.

CHAPTER 5

Shades of (Unacceptable) Behavior
Call It What It Is!

To take power away from something, you must call it by its name.

—Goethe

The impact of those who say nothing is grossly underrated. Passive onlookers and witnesses unwittingly become non-verbal, compliant supporters. Their presence of body and absence of voice serves to reinforce bullying behaviors. Studies have shown that passive observers will "spread the word that this bully is powerful, and thereby enhance the power that the bully has" (Randall, 1997).

Belonging and the Zone of Discomfort

By doing nothing, you unwittingly join the bullying culture. And, while no one would consciously choose to be complicit, the need to belong and be accepted by our peers or institutions frequently overrides the desire to do the right thing. There are several incidents where nurses were expelled from their programs. Some nurses report being told to "stay in your lane" or "get with the program"—both highly effective silencing mechanisms.

The following incident related by a third year resident further illustrates the point.

The patient was screaming in pain as the doctor performed the episiotomy because he didn't numb her first with a local anesthetic. When I commented, he responded arrogantly, "Just give her some ketamine and she'll forget about the whole thing." My parents sacrificed a lot for my education and I have to pass this rotation. I felt so helpless.

The behaviors we identify below are quite commonplace yet are **completely unacceptable** examples in contrast to the appropriate professional behaviors discussed in **Chapter Two**. The most important thing to remember is that it is **not** okay to accept, ignore or tolerate these behaviors in any way. They have a name: *horizontal hostility.*

All of the following examples are from feedback provided to the authors by practicing nurses in the field. Note that all of these behaviors are basic human responses to perceived or actual threats. No nurse thinks, *"I am going to roll my eyes now, and then turn away."* These are ALL reptilian responses that occur under stress when our neural pathways are activated by fear or a sense of threat. They're biological reactions that happen as neurons are diverted from the frontal cortex to the amygdala.

Rarely do these behaviors exist in isolation. People practicing sabotage, undermining, or intimidation, for example, may dive deep into the unacceptable behavior pool, presenting a combination of verbal and non-verbal behaviors that truly create a "zone of discomfort."

Unacceptable Behaviors

None of the following verbal and non-verbal behaviors are characteristic of a professional nurse. Let's look at these in order of most obvious to most subtle behaviors.

Yelling (Verbal)

If your ears were ringing after the conversation, then yelling was likely involved. Raised voices are unprofessional.

I was yelled at when I could not tell the nurse I was following why the IV pump was beeping.

Blaming (Verbal)

Brené Brown, 2014, states, *"Blaming is a way to discharge fear and discomfort."*

Blaming indiscriminately shifts the attention or focus to someone else. It is a strategy used to deflect responsibility and accountability. The target can be anyone. The purpose is to create or increase the credibility of the blamer while decreasing the reputation of another by finding fault or criticizing.

> *I feel belittled when there is miscommunication between the nursing assistant, the nurse, and myself as a student, and the vital signs or a dressing change does not get done and the blame is always put on the student.*

> *While working as a CNA, one of my patients fell and got injured. In the RCA meeting it was questioned why the bed alarm was not engaged.*

> *The nurse in charge of the patient pointed her finger at me and said that she didn't know why the aide didn't have the bed alarm on.*

Put-Downs (Verbal)

If you feel that you have been put-down, pay attention to the feeling. Honor it and validate it by having a conversation. Put-downs are remarks "intended to humiliate or criticize" (Oxford Dictionary, 2007).

> *I was assigned to a nurse in a SICU. I introduced myself properly and tried to help by documenting the vital signs on the flow sheet, but she made me uncomfortable. Finally, she said, "I prefer to work at my own rhythm" and then she began ignoring me.*

Name-Calling (Verbal)

Abusive language or insults (Oxford Dictionary, 2007).

You're just a young, dumb kid and you're never going to make it.

The two-year nurses are not real nurses.

Gossip (Verbal)

Gossip is a poison with multiple, frequently unpredictable, unstoppable actions, and an unfortunately long half-life. It is an uncomplimentary repetition, exaggeration, or fabrication of a story or event, regarding somebody other than the tale-bearer, in the absence of the person who is being discussed. There is no definition that sets this action in a positive light; no philosophical text that endorses it as anything other than a destructive, erosive choice. It is a malicious act because it carries the insidious purpose of demeaning, slandering or tarnishing a reputation – yet the gossiper does not perceive the damage. Gossip is a persistent struggle in healthcare for two reasons:

1. The training nurses receive reinforces and rewards the act of gathering information. The question, *"Did you know...?"* instantly gets our attention. Knowledge is a cornerstone in the world of nursing, and passing knowledge through story is a common practice as it sets the information in the mind of the speaker, and makes the listening more palatable. So, gossip contains two prongs: the act of *speaking* and the act of *listening*.

2. People gossip to remind themselves of the rules that bind them (Haidt, 2012) and to increase their social value. When we have 'the goods' on someone, we have more *perceived* power so gossip is a common way for people with low self-esteem to elevate their worth in a group.

Often managers find themselves faced with staff members who want to complain about each other, couched in the phrase, "*I have a concern about X.*" The first question from any manager needs to be, "*Have you discussed this with X?*" If so, and an equitable solution was not found, it may be time to intervene as a mediator. If not, the discussion needs to end. A savvy leader does not listen to gossip, but rather acts as a resource to offer guidance or coaching. Otherwise, the "*Nothing about me, without me*" rule applies.

Gossip is a warning sign that a larger issue exists, one that will impact patient care (Longhurst, 2016). Some managers report reliance on their 'gossips' because it keeps them apprised of what is really happening on their unit. There is a lack of professional trust that needs to be addressed and repaired if this is your methodology as good teams are transparent. Also, if this person is bringing you information, they are also taking information from you back to other staff members – regardless of the promise of confidentiality.

Infighting (Verbal)

The American Heritage College Dictionary defines infighting as, "contentious rivalry or disagreement among members of a group or organization." Working in such an environment takes a heavy toll on nurses. Constant negative comments decrease morale, rapidly drain our emotional and psychic energy, and take our focus away from the patient.

Often you will find that only a few people on a unit have a reputation for stirring up trouble, yet their continuous spewing of negative comments overrides any attempts at civility.

Evening shift is mad with day shift because they want the same staffing. The charge nurse changed the assignment and said, "I know who likes to work with whom."

Scapegoating (Verbal)

The concept of the scapegoat is an ancient one steeped in ritual. One of these rituals involved an entire community placing their "sins" on the head of a goat. The animal was then chased into the wilderness (Perera, 1986).

Nursing sees both sides of this ritual acted out when one person is repetitively blamed for an event or series of events. The profession of nursing makes this easy, as individual accountability, rather than collective responsibility, for patient care is an accepted standard. The net effect of scapegoating is to drive an individual from the ranks, even without any conscious plan to do so.

Initially, any mistake made is criticized. Eventually, the criticisms become increasingly personal and are linked to substandard performance (Hannah, 2006). Once the individual is gone, however, the ritual continues, as it, like other forms of horizontal violence, becomes embedded into the social culture of a unit or department.

Last week, a patient fell while attempting to retrieve a warm blanket. She injured her wrist in the fall, necessitating surgery. Scapegoating a single staff nurse, Maria, the other nurses complained to their manager that "Maria never puts the blankets in the warmer" and then they assigned motives to her behavior, saying it was "because she is too focused on leaving at the end of her shift instead of ensuring everything is stocked for the on-coming shift." They also say "she does not round on her patients on a regular basis." The goal is to blame the occurrence on Maria, causing her dismissal, even when the other nurses know these things are either an exaggeration, or completely untrue.

Backstabbing (Verbal)

Backstabbing is attacking someone unfairly, especially in an underhanded, deceitful manner. The goal of this behavior is to damage or destroy the reputation of a colleague, or even have them fired (Briles, 2007). These Individuals are often referred to as "two-faced," as they're known for cultivating friendships only to exploit them.

She pretended to be my friend, and so I shared my life with her. I shared my past struggles with alcoholism. But when it was time for a promotion I learned that she went to the manager and told her that I should not be promoted because I was an alcoholic.

My preceptor told me everything was fine and that I had done a good job that week. She then went to our manager saying I was "clinically not there yet." So I showed up on Monday happy and ready to learn more, only to be pulled into my manager's office and shown a long list of concerns.

Rudeness (Verbal, Non-Verbal)

Rudeness is often a social education deficit. It is affected by generations as well as culture and upbringing. For example, generally one would not feel rude for not looking a nurse in the eye or knowing his or her name because this is acceptable learned behavior. The best approach is to ask, *"Did you intend to be rude?"*

My first day working with a preceptor during transition, she was rude and then said, "Well, you know that nurses eat their young don't you?" Then she acted like I was her servant and directed me to do things while she sat at her computer and said, "Oh, I have a student to do that for me."

I answered the call light for a patient and was greeted with, "Excuse me, but I need a real nurse." The patient just wanted to go to the bathroom.

Eye-Rolling (Non-Verbal)

The most common form of horizontal hostility is eye-rolling and raised eyebrows. Historically, without an assertive voice, nurses learned to speak with their eyes and facial muscles. Healthcare workers (physicians, administrators, nurses) are all predominantly self-silencing. This is a sign of contempt and dislike. The effect of others rolling their eyes at you is that you feel insulted and disrespected. Because there are no words and the negative message is clear, people rarely respond. Here is an example provided by a student nurse:

When we walk onto the floor every Saturday morning, the nurses roll their eyes.

Ignoring (Non-Verbal)

Ignoring another individual is one of the most powerful forms of non-verbal communication known. It is also insidious, as those who are confronted with this type of behavior are likely to respond, *"Oh, I just didn't hear (see) you."*

To be ignored is to be invalidated, both as an individual and as a prospective member of a new group. Furthermore, the inability to rely on colleagues when caring for patients creates a sense of isolation and as such is detrimental to patient safety (Walrafen, Brewer, & Mulvenon, 2012). This is what one student had to say about being ignored:

For a nurse to tell me she wasn't going to allow me to do anything because I was just a student was insulting and hurtful. The entire day she barely spoke to me.

Favoritism (Non-Verbal, Verbal)

Favoritism is an open display of partiality toward certain individuals in a group by a leader. A leader gives approval or favors that are not based on merit, but rather based on his or her frequently hidden agenda (e.g., be my informer or come in when I am desperate and you won't have to work weekends). It is treatment that is abusive, unfair, or harmful.

> *Every nurse works every other weekend except for Sue. She does the schedule for the manager and is her pet so she only works every third weekend.*

> *There is definitely favoritism shown by my instructor to students she had previously. I'm just planning on keeping my head down, working hard, and counting the days until graduation.*

Cliques (Non-Verbal, Verbal)

Defined as a small, exclusive group of friends or associates, cliques are generally recognized by their extreme reluctance to include anyone new. In extreme cases, a clique will actually pride themselves on their ability to exclude others.

The following story, which you may remember from Chapter 3, is devastating and represents the level of harm and dysfunction nurses experience when cliques exist on a unit.

> *We lost a baby last night on L&D—rough night. I've been on the unit for just about six months and heard the charge nurse say, "Let's go out for breakfast." But when I asked her where we were going she turned to me, paused and said, "We don't know yet" with raised eyebrows. I got the message.*

> *No matter what I did or said or how hard I tried, they just wouldn't let me in.*

Withholding Information (Verbal, Non-Verbal)

Of all the types of horizontal violence encountered, this one has the highest potential for both nurse and patient harm. Critical information is intentionally withheld from a nurse, often because another nurse wants to see how they will react or respond, or even if they will discover the information themselves. This could range from patient allergy information, dietary preferences, or even a patient diagnosis.

The charge nurse didn't tell the emergency room nurse that a level 1 trauma patient with multiple injuries and internal wounds was inbound. She said, "Let's see what she is made of."

Undermining Activities (Non-Verbal, Verbal)

Undermining is a strategy some people with low self-esteem use because they believe it will cast them in a more positive light, even though the behavior is at the expense of a colleague's reputation. As a new nurse, this is particularly damaging in the new graduate/preceptor relationship.

Undermining jeopardizes any collegial relationship, generally causing erosion over time. It causes frustration and discouragement, and can lead a new graduate nurse to become disillusioned about the entire profession (King-Jones, 2011).

My preceptor and I had our end-of-shift debrief, as was our custom for the past four weeks. She told me everything was fine, I was progressing as expected, which was what she had been telling me after every shift. I wondered if this was really the case, because I had so many questions! I was excited to be working with this team, and wanted to believe I really was progressing. The next morning, the manager called me into her office and had a list of complaints from my preceptor, among them that I asked too many questions, which indicated to her I was unwilling to do any research.

Even though I continued working with that preceptor through my orientation, I never asked her another question; I didn't feel I could trust her. That experience made me wonder if there was anyone on that unit I could trust.

The nurse told me to crush the meds and put them into the applesauce to get them into the patient. The wife came and she was furious and told me not to feed her husband like he was a child despite my attempts to explain. Then I heard my precepting nurse in the hall say to the wife, "Well, I wouldn't have done it that way."

Intimidation (Non-Verbal, Verbal)

Intimidation is marked by fear. Often this fear is about having a discussion or sharing an idea because of the potential of ridicule, or being publicly humiliated. You feel your energy shrinking as someone bristles, overpowers, or bullies you. Animals cower, hide, run, put their heads down, or avert their eyes. Humans usually freeze and keep silent until the person leaves. They then do everything they can to avoid the intimidator in the future, as you can imagine would be the case in the following examples.

The nursing instructor began by saying, "No one will get an A in this class. Possibly 17% may get a B and the majority will be lucky to pass. Any questions?"

I was working in an ICU, and came on shift to see I had been given three patients, when we are only supposed to have two. All three of them were mechanically ventilated, and on a number of medications. I asked my charge nurse if we could change this, because I was uncomfortable with that assignment. She yelled at me, "What do you mean you are uncomfortable taking this assignment? I spent an hour trying to divide this up fairly, and all you can do is complain! If you are not capable of doing what is expected of you, then maybe you should not be working on this unit!"

Sabotage (Non-Verbal, Verbal)

Sabotage is defined as "treacherous action to defeat or hinder a cause or an endeavor; deliberate subversion" (American Heritage College Dictionary, 2007). What makes it so devastating is that there is **intention** behind the act of a colleague; this is not an accidental act. In a sabotage situation, you are set up to fail. Here are some examples of sabotage:

I was looking all over the floor for a pulse oximetry unit and I asked the nurse at the desk if she knew where one was. My patient was a fresh post op and I needed to get the oxygen level. She said "No, haven't seen one." Ten minutes later I watched as she opened the drawer in front of her and took out the pulse ox for her patient.

My clinical instructor belittled us every day we were at the hospital. She walked around saying, "I can fail you." She would hide my medications as I scanned them so when we did our final count, the med wasn't there.

I was involved in treating a pediatric asthma patient, and had several things to get done. An experienced nurse came into the room and asked if she could help. Initially, I was relieved, and asked if she could assemble the nebulizer unit for the Albuterol while I finished the intravenous line and administered another medication. When I completed that task, I turned around to see the nebulizer unit sitting on the mayo stand, in pieces. I heard her at the nurses' station announcing that I did not know how to assemble this very simple piece of equipment. Fortunately, the respiratory therapist arrived at that moment; he noticed a central piece was missing from the nebulizer assembly and commented to me, "Nobody could put this together without that piece." We stabilized the patient, and when I reflected on what had happened, I just felt sick.

Now You Know

- Lateral violence is undermining the entire profession of nursing.

- It is implicated in the current nursing shortage.

- None of the forms of horizontal violence are acceptable.

- These behaviors are unethical: The American Nurses Association sites any form of horizontal violence as unethical practice (Lachman, 2015).

- If you would like to learn more, follow this link: Incivility, Bullying and Workplace Violence. ANA Position Statement. *www.nursingworld.org/MainMenuCategories/Workplace Safety/Healthy-Nurse/bullyingworkplaceviolence*

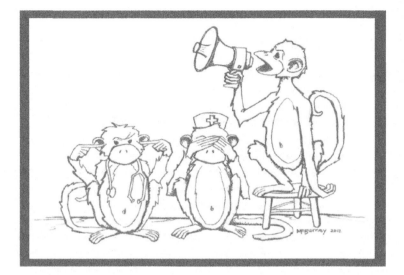

Nothing about me, without me

CHAPTER 6

Choosing Your Role in a Hostile Work Environment

Ouch!

> *If you are neutral in situations of injustice, you have chosen the side of the oppressor.*
>
> —Desmond Tutu

If as nurses we are in fear, then our patients are in danger. There is a significant body of research that clearly states the impact of rude behaviors on our ability to deliver safe quality care to our patients. Rude behaviors make us physically sick, distract us from our patients, create moral distress, increase sick days, foster fear and self-doubt, and lower our self-esteem and confidence. It's easy to imagine a student nurse's reaction to the following:

> *Her clinical instructor grabbed her by the shoulders reprimanding her as the staff nurses looked on. Unfortunately, the students who experience this type of abuse really feel as if they have no recourse. We are afraid to say anything for fear of being kicked out of the program, especially if the clinical instructor happens to be friends with the department chair! So we cry, we vent, we curse, we vomit, and we try to get through the program one day at a time. Where is the student advocate?*

If you randomly collected a hundred stories as we did, you wouldn't need to read the research. The stories from student nurses clearly demonstrate the impact of working in a hostile environment.

What's a Hostile Work Environment?

Any nurse who is "crying, venting, vomiting, and cursing" is *extremely* upset. Rude and hostile interactions have a profound impact on how we feel and, therefore, on the quality of care we are able to deliver. If nurses don't communicate for fear of retribution or ridicule, the patients we are caring for pay the consequences, up to and including death (Maxfield, Grenny, Lavandero, & Groah, 2010).

When humans are upset, their brains automatically ignite a flight or fight response. These negative interactions physically rewire our neural circuitry from the frontal cortex to the amygdala. This is the oldest, most reptilian part of the brain—not the best place to be coming from as you titrate a dopamine drip, calculate the right amount for a pediatric patient, or apply critical thinking skills to evaluate lab results.

Furthermore, nursing is known as a *tacit knowledge* profession. You learn by building your practice and applying that knowledge repetitively and having it validated by more experienced peers. It's historical and evidenced-based.

Lateral violent behavior interrupts this process of learning.

Choosing Your Role

Nursing is rewarding yet stressful work. This stress can be minimized by a great team, or intensified by a bad one. Even after a stressful day you can leave work feeling great if you have a supportive team. It is an incredible feeling to be a part of something larger than yourself.

Like the middle-school playground, there are many roles where emotions rule and commotion abounds—witness, victim, and bully. Deciding not to take the role of the bully is not enough. Each of these roles plays a part in lateral violence, and each is detrimental to the healthy workplace. **Don't play a part.**

The Role of Witness

There is no such thing as an innocent bystander. Do you ever hear people talking about someone when they are not present? If so, then we guarantee you that they are talking about you when you are not there. Never stand by and listen to gossip. Adopt this mantra:

Nothing about me, without me

Gossip Triage Tool

What are some healthy alternatives to gossiping when you want to belong and be accepted?

1. Walk away.

2. Ask yourself:

   - Is the person being discussed present?
   - What thought, feeling or previous incident has made it more comfortable for me to speak *about* them rather than *to* them directly?
   - How can I improve the relationship so that I am bringing issues or concerns to others the same way I would like them to bring issues to my attention?

3. Say something, such as:

   - *I don't feel right talking about ____ when they are not here. Let's wait until they can be included in the conversation.*
   - *It looks like you and ____ need to have a conversation, but ____ is not here.*
   - *I am uncomfortable listening to this because I wouldn't want anyone talking behind my back and I try to treat others the same.*

The Role of Bully

But what if you see someone yelling, sabotaging, undermining, belittling, or degrading one of your peers? This person is using one, two, or more of the unacceptable behaviors from Chapter 5 to harm a coworker. What do you do in that situation?

You have two options when dealing with bullies:

1. Do nothing (no scruples). See the link to the Fousey Bullying Experiment: *youtube.com/watch?v=EisZTB4ZQxY*

2. Do something (scruples: a spine, morals, or a conscience).

Imagine your nurse manager, mother, or child is standing right next to you. Is this appropriate behavior? Speak up and begin by approaching the perpetrator with, *"May I speak to you for a moment in private?"*

Go to a private place (for example, a soiled utility room). This gives them time to calm down and focus. Begin with *"I am concerned... worried..."* Explain the impact of their behavior and ask them to stop.

Alternatively, approach both nurses and say, *"For the safety of our patients, this must stop."*

The Role of Victim

You are not alone—unfortunately. Many have walked into a trap set by peers who feel compelled to put them down so that they can feel better about themselves. And you are not imagining it.

> *We believe you.*
> *We believe you.*
> *We believe you.*

Yes, we need a Dr. Phil for healthcare, as most likely this is the way many nurses were treated. But now that you know that hostility is a social and primal behavior of human herds, let's talk about how to make it better, and why it matters so much.

Building a Better Work Environment

Dr. Cynthia Clark (2013) created a progressive continuum of uncivil behaviors to illustrate how some negative behaviors may have more severe consequences than others. Left unaddressed, non-verbal behaviors such as eye-rolling may escalate to more damaging and overt behaviors such as sarcasm, racial slurs, intimidation and violence. Therefore, it's very important to stop any form of hostility.

But what if you speak up and nothing really changes? Try the D-E-S-C Conversation model.

TOOL: The D-E-S-C Model

Describe the behavior (Facts first)   D: *When...*

Explain the impact of the behavior (Story second)   E: *I feel...*

    Pause for 4 seconds

State the desired outcome (Ask for what you need)   S: *Can you...*

Consequence if behavior doesn't change or   C: *So that...*

    End with a question

    Would you be willing to...?

Here is an example of D-E-S-C in action:

I was helping a nurse on the ICU unit prepare a bed for a new admission and we were chatting. She said, "I really don't know why they hired you... it's bad enough that the more senior nurses have to deal with us who have only been nurses for a few years, but now you guys are coming and asking all sorts of dumb questions."

I stopped her and said, "I worked very hard to get to where I am today and did extremely well in my internship, so I truly believe the manager hired me because she saw I was doing exceptional work."'

She responded, "Oh no, I wasn't saying anything about you. I just don't understand why they would fill ICU positions with new grads when we need experienced nurses."

I replied, "That sounds like an issue you need to take up with someone else, not me."

The Emotional and Psychological Impact

Even though the new-to-practice nurse's responses were professional, she experienced a considerable amount of emotional fallout. She confided:

This whole interaction with this nurse really took the air out of my balloon. I went home feeling awful, like I was back in grade school and the girls didn't like me or want me around. That feeling really stinks.

For a brief moment I contemplated if I should stay on this unit. It is really amazing how a few words made me feel this way.

Let's use Control+Alt+Delete to reframe her understanding of the interaction and then map out possible new responses using D-E-S-C.

Use Control+Alt+Delete

Control: Examine the situation. Take control. Don't label someone else's intent.

I wonder why the nurse would say something like that. Maybe that's what someone said to her when she was new to the unit.

Alt: Re-examine. Consider Options. Choose a course of action.

If I stay silent, this situation will gnaw at me, and it may very likely happen again.

I could talk to her today and use the DESC model, and maybe write it down first beforehand.

Delete: Use the D-E-S-C technique to script your new responses.

Use D-E-S-C

Describe: *May I talk to you for just a moment about your last comment?*

Explain: *Because I am a new graduate, this is about me. I feel undermined and certainly not supported knowing that this is your position.*

Pause – 4 seconds

State: *I understand that questions are frustrating and time consuming in a busy ICU. Yet I cannot imagine that you got to where you are without asking questions.*

Conclusion/Question: *Will you treat me the way you wanted to be received when you came here?*

Success Tips

- Always try to handle interpersonal problems directly with the person involved. In nursing some challenging responses have been:

- *I don't have a problem. It's your problem.*

- *I don't have time.*

- *Don't worry about it. Everything's fine.* (But it isn't.)

- These responses are spoken by people because they have always worked to push others away. Remember, the purpose of their response is to silence you (as I am sure they have silenced others in the past).

- Write it out. It helps to put your thoughts down on paper. Take time to think about your experience, how you felt, and what you need. Don't forget the "Ask."

- Begin with, *"May I talk to you for a minute in private?"* If they say no, propose another time.

- Remember to be aware of your emotions. If you are angry, hateful, and mad, all these emotions will sabotage the conversation by making the other person afraid.

- If you're unable to resolve the situation yourself, ask the manager to help coach you or mediate, but don't ever go to the manager's office complaining about another person who is not present.

Now You Know

- If you are upset, your patients are in danger.

- You now have a set of reliable tools: The D-E-S-C is a communication tool for your tool-kit, as well as Control+Alt+Delete and the related Construct/Deconstruct.

- There is more than one actor in the hostility play: the witness, victim, and the bully each play a part. Don't take on any of the roles in this drama. Adults solve their own problems with other adults.

- Gossip is a culture killer: Remember the phrase, *"Nothing about me without me."* Never go to your manager without the person you are having a problem with.

- If you don't practice scenarios ahead of time, you won't use them when you need them the most.

CHAPTER 7

Preparing Yourself with Cognitive Rehearsal

What Do I Do Again?

Bad boys, bad boys, whatcha gonna do? Whatcha gonna do when they come for you?

—Inner Circle

In this chapter, we'll build on the skills you've learned in earlier chapters, including Control+Alt+Delete and the D-E-S-C Communication Model. Here, we're going to give you the keys to another great assertive communication tool: *Cognitive Rehearsal.* With cognitive rehearsal, you gain the advantage of knowing how to react and what to say whenever unacceptable behavior rears its ugly head.

Scripts work! For the parents reading this chapter, you may also find cognitive rehearsal helpful when facing the thirty-fifth time your darling child has exhibited a particular undesirable behavior. For example, how do you remind a child not to try to eat an entire plate of spaghetti in one bite? (You might develop a script like this: *If it doesn't fit on your fork, it isn't going to fit in your mouth.*)

Cognitive Rehearsal

Nurses who can handle confrontations decrease their rate of burnout and stress. Cognitive Rehearsal (CR) is having a pre-learned expression in your head designed by you to respond to ambiguous and/or upsetting situations. It can be a script, or an expression you're familiar with. When you've got your set of CR tools, you're ready for anything.

CR is a skill set for today's nurse. It offers the antidote to ruminating, complaining, whining about a situation, being passive, and never speaking to the person you're upset with directly. CR has been proven to help nurses build up a strong resilience to the negative impact of harmful words or behaviors (Griffin, 2006, 2014), (Stagg, 2011).

The Rules of Cognitive Rehearsal

When you handle confrontations, you increase your own self-confidence and set the expectation that you're a person who speaks their truth and can be trusted. You establish your reputation as someone who will speak directly to a person if they have a problem or concern. This fact alone dramatically increases trust. The goal is to make it known to the person that the behavior is not okay with you.

General Rule #1

Always ask to speak to a person in private, because audiences affect the behavior of the person you're speaking with—it is the professional thing to do. Your first phrase to have ready is the following:

May I speak to you in private for a minute?

The possible responses to your question are yes, no, or why. Let's look at the responses you can have at the ready if the person says anything other than yes. It is absolutely critical that you are prepared for any response.

General Rule #2

Speak up. Say what you see. Point out the behavior.

I noticed that you rolled your eyes when you picked up the assignment sheet.

Always validate your interpretation.

Did that mean that you thought the assignment I made was unfair?

Possible Outcome: Challenging You with WHY

You may experience pushback in the form of a challenge to your valid question.

For example, your colleague might respond with an angry tone, saying, *"What do you need to speak to me in private for? I don't have anything to say to you that anyone else can't hear."*

People who behave this way are insecure, have low self-esteem, and seek safety in audiences. Your tone of voice and non-verbal behavior is absolutely critical in this situation. If necessary, you can give them a guarantee with the following proven request:

> *Will you stay in a conversation with me until we both feel alright?*

Having this sort of response at the ready is important because, in the United States, confronting and conversations have been historically hierarchical and one-way: *"I will tell you what I think and feel—and then we're done."*

This one-way meme is an unhealthy, subtle, yet powerful undercurrent in our society. It abdicates our personal responsibility. Possible inviting responses you can have ready are:

> *It only involves you and me, so I want to keep it private.*

> *No, I really need for us to have a conversation now, and we can't do that publicly because I respect you and want to avoid gossip.*

> *This is how professional nurses communicate their concerns.*

Possible Outcome: They Say NO

So maybe someone will not speak to you, or flat out says "NO." What do you do?

Bump it up. Move to a higher level. Reinforce the need for a private conversation by using CR, with phrases like the following:

I've been taught to go directly to the person I want to speak to rather than the manager. Would you prefer I talk to someone else about this?

I really wish that we could talk because I know that we can resolve this ourselves.

In the absence of cooperative communication, leadership must be informed. If you cannot get someone to speak with you, then ask the manager to mediate the situation and be present. Never run to the manager expecting him or her to solve your personal communication issues before you've tried to resolve them yourself. Conversations are the building blocks of professional relationships.

Addressing Lateral Violence with Cognitive Rehearsal

We've discussed lateral violence in every chapter of this book. You know the behaviors: eye-rolling, sighing, raised eyebrows, sucking in air, chuckling, being shown "the hand," ignoring, intimidation, cliques, and favoritism, etc. The following are some CR scripts that you can adapt to fit your own experiences.

Ignoring

Ignoring is when you feel excluded from a conversation that you feel you should have been included in; for example, a change in practice that no one shared with you or nurses talking about your patient. As close to the time that this happens, you should have a private conversation focused on the behavior.

Example: You witness two nurses talking about your assigned patient. Address the person you hear speaking directly by saying:

Can I speak with you for a moment in the lounge? (Seek privacy.)

Are you aware that I have Mrs. Jones today? (Validating, because maybe they genuinely didn't know!)

I feel uncomfortable when I am not included in conversations about my patient. (Observe the response.)

Response: Their response will guide you to what is next. Let's look at those options:

Option A: They're defensive.

Defuse. Seek to take any emotional charge out of this situation. If you show that you're not attacking them, they will feel safe enough to continue a professional conversation. For example, apologize by saying:

I didn't know you had that patient. I am sorry.

Option B: They're mean and sarcastic.

They say, *"You should already know what is going on with your own patient."*

You respond by redirecting the focus:

Your tone sounds mean and unprofessional. Let's keep this conversation at a higher level.

Can you help me understand how I did not get this important information?

What you're doing here is defusing, redirecting, and not playing the game. When you ask for help you once again level the playing field. Asking for assistance requires humility and a firm commitment to knowing the truth—integrity. These are the qualities of a truly professional nurse—a dauntless nurse.

Option C: Gossip.

A nursing assistant tells you that the other nurses are talking about your patient.

Never act on secondhand information. Validate by going to see what is happening and only react to what you see or hear personally. Third party information leads your unit down a path where the manager is listening to gossip about you. Follow this valuable rule, which you may remember from Chapter 6: *Nothing about me, without me.*

Intimidation

It's all about the pecking order. Dogs growl, cats hiss, porcupines bristle, and humans *intimidate*. Intimidation is the way that humans maintain their pecking order and respond to perceived threats. It's how we herd people in and out of groups. The behavior is probably more operationalized than we realize.

We often do not see these behaviors at our own level, but can easily see them in people who have perceived power over us. For example, physicians can intimidate with tactics such as a loud voice, lack of eye contact, and ignoring. Then nurses who have observed these behaviors adopt them without realizing it. Or intimidation can be perfectly still and silent—a feeling you sense. So what do you do?

- Don't put your tail between your legs. Rule number one: *Maintain eye contact.*

- Don't puff up, growl, or hiss. This will escalate the situation. Instead, initiate a professional conversation that always begins with asking to see someone in private.

Example: As a new-to-practice nurse, you ask a question and the nurse responds with, *"So where did you go to school again?"* or *"How many years have you been a nurse?"*

Clearly, these responses feel intimidating. What do you say?

- In the moment, with witnesses: Answer the question.

- In a private conversation: *I felt bad today about something you said, and wanted to talk to you about it. When I asked you a question, you responded by asking me where I went to school. I felt less-than, in an awkward spot and confused. Were you inferring that I should have known this information? My goal is to establish a relationship where I can ask questions, validate my knowledge, and acquire more. But your comment shut me down.*

Favoritism

Favoritism is a perception. It is comprised of observing unfair behaviors or practices. For example, the nurse who always picks up the extra shifts, seems to never take patients on isolation precautions, or routinely comes in late to work.

Favoritism can be real or imagined. So you have to validate. Here is how:

- Collect the data.
- Identify the trade-off.
- Point out the unfair practices.

The first person you should address is NOT the manager or charge nurse, but always **the individual** because that is what we all prefer. If this is not successful, then you can move up the chain of command.

Cliques

We've discussed cliques in other chapters because they are common and always problematic. They are more obscure than favoritism, but still need to be addressed because if you have cliques, then you DON'T have a team. For example, cliques don't exist in *The Blue Angels* or *The Boston Celtics.* Cliques divide the precious focus and energy of any group. They exist because at one time in the history of the group, people felt unsafe and the need for protection.

Like all of our advice, this isn't about you. It's about human behavior in groups. Another primary function is that they raise the low self-esteem of the clique's members. People feel more important when they belong to something exclusive.

1. Decide how much time it will take you to be accepted by this group. Then add 2-3 more months because you're in nursing. Be patient.

2. Observe to determine who the informal leader of the group is. In private, ask them what you have to do to belong. This act alone may be the gate- way to inclusion. (They will be surprised at your question because these behaviors are unconscious. Remember middle school?)

3. If, after a significant period of time you never feel accepted in a group, move on. Cliques are reason enough to quit a job because you will be constantly sapped of psychic energy and strength. Professional nurses work as a team—synchronous, sharing knowledge, giving advice, and inclusive of everyone for the benefit of the patient. When you work in this type of environment you feel incredibly empowered. Every nurse, especially new nurses, deserve this.

Rudeness

Researchers have proven that simply witnessing rude behavior in the workplace "significantly impairs our ability to perform cognitive tasks" (Porath and Erez, 2007). This is because we are human. Observing or experiencing rudeness shifts our neurological wiring swiftly to the amygdala, leaving us distracted and needing to recover. This puts our patients in serious danger.

A good nurse is **never** rude. Rudeness is not only toxic, but contagious (Huffington Post, 7/28/15). Rudeness can be covert or overt, as shown in the following examples:

- Working with someone for years but never learning their names.

- Making personal comments.

- Making inappropriate jokes.

- Prying inappropriately into personal matters, sharing too much personal info.

- Exhibiting rude, disrespectful, or discourteous behaviors.

What do you do?

- Ask to speak to the person in private.

- Describe the behavior and its effect on you.

Example: Mary arrived late for her shift and then started demanding that her assignment should be changed. You're a new nurse and have the same patients as yesterday, yet the charge nurse begins changing the assignment. What do you say?

Ask to speak to the charge nurse in private first. Speak your truth:

> *I know you worked hard to make a consistent assignment so that I could have the best clinical experience possible. I am asking you not to change it when pressured or bullied. Can I please keep the patients I had yester- day? I have my plan of care completed for all of them.*

Scapegoating

The purpose of targeting or creating a scapegoat is to draw attention away from the people who are doing it, and to create a fall guy, so the position has been filled. This increases the psychological safety of any vulnerable group with low self-esteem.

Undermining Activities, Sabotage, and Withholding Information

Examples: A bad schedule or assignment, refusing to help, pretending not to notice when you're upset or overworked, talking about you behind your back, setting you up to fail with a bad report or not relaying critical lab values, wrong instruments on tray, wrong preference card in OR, or phone calls, writing you up for poor charting, etc.

If you feel undermined, say something. The worst thing you can do is be silent. For example, you might say:

> *Can you help me understand how this situation could have happened?* (Be as specific as possible.)

*Can you help me understand why I was not told about the
low potassium level?*

*It was my understanding that there was more information
available than meets the eye. Can you and I meet in private
and review the situation?*

*This card and case was pulled for Dr. Evans, but I needed Dr.
Simpson's. What went wrong?*

Success Tips for Professional Communication

- First, validate the facts.

- Seek privacy.

- Find the courage and commitment.

- Say what you see: *I noticed that...*

- Maintain professional composure at all times.

- Adopt the motto: *Nothing about me, without me.*

- Repeat often: *It's not about me... It's not about me...*

Now You Know

- Cognitive rehearsal means having prepared scripts and
  practicing them empowers you to respond. You will find a list
  of them printed out on the last page of the book. Put them in
  your badge holder or post them in your locker.

- It's not just about the words. People aren't used to assertive
  communication. But you can help your peers feel safe by
  beginning with, *"Can you stay in conversation with me until
  we both feel alright?"*

- Speaking your truth is the only way to keep our patients safe.
  A team needs every voice.

CHAPTER 8

Dauntless Trailblazers

Confidence Builders

> *Every man must be his own leader.*
> *He now knows enough not to follow other people.*
> *He must follow the light that's within himself,*
> *And through this light, he will create a new community.*

> — Laurens Van der Post

In this chapter you'll learn from the experiences of other nurses and nurse leaders who have incorporated the use of D-E-S-C, Ctrl+Alt+Delete, and Cognitive Rehearsal into their day-to-day conversations which are the building blocks of our profession. Remember: *Power=Voice.*

D-E-S-C in Action

Imagine *yourself* in the following real-life scenarios and practice how to respond using the communication tools you have acquired. By practicing responses to difficult situations, you will be more confident in speaking up to stop negative verbal and non-verbal behavior and will help create a more positive culture in your own workplace.

#1 Ignoring

Margo is a brand new nurse and this is her first day on the job. In very subtle ways, her preceptor has sent the message that she in the way. There is no time to even ask a question and Margo is constantly running to catch up with her preceptor.

May I speak with you for a minute in private?

Describe: *I noticed today that you seemed bothered by my questions and I felt in the way.*

Explain: *I understand that your workload is heavy, but when you ignore me, I feel unimportant and I am getting the message that you wish I wasn't here.*

State: *I really need to find some time to connect with you. Could we meet at the beginning, middle and end of the shift for just five minutes to give me an opportunity to ask questions so I can learn?*

Consequence: *I really want to be the best nurse that I can be, and I learn best when I have an opportunity to stop and think and absorb information.*

#2 Gossip, Blaming and Put-downs

Bill was late for report one day. As he opened the door he heard Margaret say, *"I hate following Bill because he always leaves things for me to do."*

After report was over, Bill asked, *"Margaret, can I talk to you for a minute in private?"*

Describe: *When I opened the door to the report room, I heard you say that you hate following me because I leave things undone and dump on the next shift.*

Explain: *I was really upset when I heard that because I would never intentionally leave work undone.*

State: *What I need is the information that you have that will help me be successful and be thought of as a team player.*

Consequence: *My goal is to hear you say how much you like to follow me because everything is in order, but clearly you have information I need to make that happen.*

Or: *Could you please write down the things you are finding on a sticky note so that I have the information I need to succeed?*

Or: *If you think I am not doing my fair share of the work, please discuss it with me directly.*

#3 Undermining

Jose is an experienced flight nurse who has moved to another city and accepted a job in the local emergency room. If there is a serious event, the code is "TRIAGE, TRIAGE." The charge nurse asked Jose to watch a sleeping patient when shortly afterward he heard this code. Quickly he responded to find a man leaning over the counter, clutching his chest and sweating – clearly a heart attack. Everything went well – except for the next day when he was called into the manager's office and was reprimanded for "not doing as you are told' because the charge nursed complained to the manager.

Describe: *Thank you for sharing the concerns of the charge nurse with me.*

Explore: *It is upsetting to learn that rather than talk to me directly, the charge nurse felt the need to involve you.*

State: *In the future, if someone has a problem that concerns me, I would appreciate your inviting me into the conversation, or redirecting them to handle the issue with me as we are all adults.*

Consequence: *Because we cannot have the highly functioning team we need to care for our patients if we don't have the skill and courage to talk to each other when conflicts arise.*

#4 Put-downs and Gossip

Laura is a newly hired registered nurse who has just completed her Associate of Nursing Program. She has only been at this new ambulatory surgery center for a month when she notices that she is always working with the same person. She asks to be reassigned to get more experience in other operating rooms. Later that same day, she overhears Sarah, a circulating nurse say, *"I don't have anything against her...it's just that I only want to work with real nurses."*

Sarah, can I talk to you for a minute in private?

Describe: *I overheard you say that you only wanted to work with 'real' nurses.*

Explore: *I am a real nurse. I passed the same NCLEX as all the others to become a registered nurse, and was upset to hear you infer that I was less than capable. Perhaps you have had experiences like that in the past?*

State: *I would sincerely appreciate your giving me a chance before jumping to the conclusion that I cannot measure up to the caliber of nurse you expect, because I too have the same high standard and I want to work with people just like you.*

Consequence: *So I would appreciate you giving me a chance, sharing where you see I can improve, and supporting me to that end. What do you think? Will you please give me a chance to work with you?*

#5 Rudeness and Intimidation

The new trauma surgeon in the ICU has an attitude problem. Every single encounter has left Maria feeling "less than". When she called with important patient information, he acts bothered. When she reported a critical lab value, he responded, *"I already know that".*

Doctor, can I speak to you for a minute in private?

Describe: *I would like to talk to you about yesterday when you I gave you the critically low hematocrit value and you responded with, "I already know that."*

Explore: *That is the third time I have brought you important patient information only to be dismissed, and it feels bad and is* embarrassing. *The impact is that not only I, but others, will eventually stop notifying you or hesitate to call you.*

State: *This break in communication could have devastating effects on our patients. In the future, I would appreciate it if you would say 'thank you'.*

Consequence: *This will help continue our culture of teamwork, professionalism and collegiality that supports our patients.*

Control+Alt+Delete Scenarios

#1 Ignoring

Edossa called out sick last week due to the flu that she caught from her toddler, after having to call out sick the week before to take care of her sick children. Now every time she walks into a place where the nurses are gathered, she gets the silent treatment. She feels an awkwardness in the air that just wasn't there before.

Control: I am picking up vibes that are uncomfortable.

Alt: I wonder why people are upset with me.

Maybe people are upset with my calling out sick so much in the last month – or maybe I did something that I don't know about.

This is not my imagination. I need to check it out.

Delete: I need to ask if they are upset that I have missed so much work and ask about the silence.

#2 Ignoring

Judy is a seasoned OR scrub nurse who has just completed setting up the instrument table for the upcoming open heart procedure. Her manager calls her out of the room saying, "I need you to help hand-assemble a tray for Dr. Jones' procedure. You're the only one here today familiar with what he uses." Since her patient isn't expected for another 15 minutes, and nobody is in the room, Judy goes to help, with her manager's assurance that she will notify the team lead of Judy's whereabouts. It takes 20 minutes to assemble the tray before Judy can return to her original room. She arrives to find the patient already on the OR table. One of the nurses is staring at her, and her team lead will not even look at her as they complete the 'time out' for the patient.

Control: Something feels really off here; this is not how my team usually acts toward me and I feel uneasy.

Alt: Did my manager let my team lead know where I was? If not, maybe they drew a wrong conclusion about why I wasn't here.

Delete: I need to ask my team lead if she got the message about my whereabouts from our manager. If not, I can succinctly explain what happened.

Cognitive Rehearsal Scripts from Dauntless Nurses

The following are vignettes of nurses who took back their power in a variety of real-life situations. Reading these stories helps to hardwire positive and professional responses. Which story resonates with you? Underline the moment in each narrative where the nurse decided to be dauntless.

#1 Non-verbal Innuendo and Raised Eyebrows, Undermining and Sabotage
CR Script: Gary's Script for Non-verbal Lateral Violence

I noticed by your facial expression that there might be something you want to say to me. It's okay to speak to me directly.

I noticed you raised your eyebrows when I made that comment.

On my unit, just one particular nurse causes 99% of all the lateral violence and negative activity. She has been spoken to, but she never takes it seriously and continues to be abusive to whomever she wants! I believe it's mostly new employees and mostly new to practice RN's. The nurse manager knows about these behaviors, but nothing changes.

I use what I've learned about lateral violence every day. So far, speaking to this individual directly about the individuals I learn best from has worked. Now she does give me feedback.

I definitely feel that she has set up situations where I've had to speak to her directly, but I'm learning to speak up for myself and the patient. At first I thought it would be awkward to use them, but after a few times, the scripts became a comfort that boosted my confidence. I'm grateful for learning some rehearsed responses as this nurse calls for trying them all!

#2 Dealing with Cliques

CR Script: Ann's Response to Cliques and Unfair Assignments

When an event happens that is contrary to that which was my understanding, it leaves me with questions. Help me understand how this situation happened.

Nurses everywhere I've worked are very clique-oriented. A "cool group" clique forms very quickly and undermines the "non-cool group." I've also found that the nurses outside the clique are assigned much harder assignments. I see them doing all the admissions and discharges, even going off floor to the pharmacy for the patients' scripts before they go home. I've also seen them assigned patients with higher levels of acuity, which translates to more work for the "non-cool" nurse.

As a direct result of these clique behaviors, I found it extremely difficult to adjust and fit in. The clique that worked my night shift treated me like an "invisible nurse." I went home most mornings crying in my car along the way. I never let them (or my family) see me cry. But I didn't want that group to get the best of me, so I was very motivated to find a solution.

I didn't know much about lateral violence, but I eventually realized that these nurses' behaviors were exactly that. I also didn't know any way to counter such behavior. I learned from a new-to-practice nurse that she had taken a class in school focusing on lateral violence and cognitive rehearsal.

I was intrigued and began to read more myself. Now I'm an expert—I've learned how to defend myself and address lateral violence when it happens to me. I now say, *"When an event happens that is contrary to that which was my understanding it leaves me with question. Help me understand how this situation happened."*

#3 Snide Remarks, Non-verbal Innuendos, Raised Eyebrows, and Face-Making

CR Script: Roger Champions Manager Training

I noticed that only staff receives the lateral violence training. Is it possible that this program could be mandatory for managers as well?

Most of the lateral violence on our unit comes from the nurse manager, who feels that it's okay to say the most ridiculous things. He starts early in the morning at first shift and says out loud, *"Nobody is working here today! I see not one body moving towards WORK, I just hear chatter, chatter, chatter."*

It's the most unprofessional thing that I've heard. He also said out loud, *"Just so you all know, I'm only hiring nurses who aren't married and don't have children so they won't call in sick. Kids are always sick!"*

I met with upper management and asked that manager level employees receive some lateral violence training, as it was only the staff level nurses who were trained and received the cognitive rehearsal cards.

#4 Lack of Respect and Gossip

CR Script: Mary's Perspective as a Second Degree, Late Entry Nurse

That sounds like information that should remain confidential. It's not right to speak about someone who isn't here.

I was older when I started nursing school and I had a career in business before going back to school to be a nurse practitioner. I heard of nurse practice lateral violence, but thought of it in a very benign way as just idle gossip. In business, though not welcome, gossip is just banter and kind of ignored, and definitely not seen as harmful.

However, when I was in nursing school and then again in my nurse practitioner program, gossip caused a great deal of angst and grief for my patients as well as my colleagues. Gossip was a definite form of disrespect but seemed like a cultural norm. In fact, one of our new primary care physicians was a victim of vicious gossip and succumbed to it by taking her own life.*

I now interpret any form of gossip as a serious lack of professionalism and have a default pre-rehearsed expression that I practice often so it can be at the tip of my tongue! I say *"That sounds like information that should remain confidential."*

* Editor's Note: In 2015, 350 physicians and 150 residents committed suicide.

#5 Making Yourself Unavailable and Withholding Information

CR Script: Mike's patient at risk

It's my understanding that there is more information about this patient. Please help me understand how I did not get the necessary pertinent information on my patient.

For the most part, the nurses on my floor are civil to each other, although some can be very rude and talk down to you. The nurses that do this are typically the more experienced ones. It seems that they feel superior and want to stay that way. They never share their general nursing knowledge, and they also won't share information on specific patients they've had—even when that patient is now assigned to you!

I saw it right away as withholding information and used the script from my cognitive rehearsal card: *It's my understanding that there is more information about this patient, help me understand.*

It really did feel good to have something to say!

Dauntless Communication Tip

We'll end this chapter with a tip provided by a dauntless nurse named Andrea, who has dealt with stress and lateral violence in interactions between the emergency department and other units. Her advice is very simple:

When you know the drama and can anticipate a repeatable situation, memorize a professional response.

Keep this advice and the definition of dauntless in the back of your mind so that you, too, can develop confident communication skills in the face of lateral violence.

---

dauntless [dawnt-lis, dahnt-les]

Synonyms: brave, intrepid, valiant, audacious, courageous

adjective **1.** not to be daunted or intimidated; fearless; intrepid; bold: a dauntless hero.

noun **2.** (initial capital letter). Also called Douglas SBD, the principal U.S. Navy fleet bomber of early World War II, capable of carrying bombs or depth charges and particularly successful as a dive bomber.

The history of the world is peopled with dauntless men and women who refused to be subdued or "tamed" by fear.

AFTERWORD

Self-Reflection

Oh, no. I've done this. Am I a bully?

This handbook covers material that is uncomfortable for a variety of reasons. Horizontal violence is one of the last taboo topics in nursing, and you may have found yourself reflecting on incidences that are painful, or conducting an unsettling self-examination. You may have read some of the material and thought, *"Oh, no. I have done this. Am I a bully?"*

Recall that in prior chapters we discussed the unconscious nature of horizontal violence—much of the behavior is learned and then mimicked in order to feel accepted. If you are reflecting on behavior you don't wish to continue or perpetuate, here are some additional questions to aid in that reflection:

1. Do your conversations with coworkers tend to be dialogues or monologues?
2. It's peer review time. When you ask coworkers to complete one for you, do they readily agree or do their replies range from saying, *"I've already done my three—sorry!"* to avoiding the topic with you at all costs?
3. Do you derive satisfaction when one of your peers fails?
4. Do your peers confide in you, seek your advice, or ask for your aid in problem solving? Or, do you find yourself learning of issues days or weeks after somebody else has addressed them, realizing you have been left out of the loop entirely?
5. When was the last time you solved a problem at work?
6. Do others describe you as *"tough?"*
7. If your facility gave a seminar on horizontal violence, would you attend? If not, would it be a matter of scheduling or do you believe you simply do not need it or are above it?
8. How would you rate your listening skills on a scale of 0-10?

9. You are in the break room and a coworker makes a disparaging comment about a peer. Do you join the conversation and contribute negative comments of your own or do you advocate for your peer and finding a better solution?

10. Your manager asks you to precept a nursing student for two weeks. Which of the following best describes your reaction?

   a. You welcome the opportunity and seek ways to make it optimal for you and your student.

   b. You grudgingly accept the assignment because it looks good on a resume.

   c. You consider it your chance to make someone else suffer as much as you did when you were a student.

The Results are in...

You may be feeling a sense of relief at this point, or you may be feeling a bit of anxiety or even shock as you recognize unacceptable patterns in your own behavior. How do you go about making amends for your behavior? Where do you begin?

The Undo Command!

 Service recovery is possible if you are serious about it. Research of horizontal violence continually demonstrates that once individuals are aware of their actions and the effect those actions are having on people around them, there is motivation for, and demonstration of, long-term change.

This research also acknowledges that nurses who realize their behavior has been consistently labeled as bullying suffer a drop in their self-esteem. Understand that this will be a process and that you deserve support, too. This support may not be available from your work peers initially, so consider other sources as you make your initial efforts.

Communication Confidence Self-Test

How Dauntless Are You?

Use this appendix as a way to test your reactions to challenging situations. The scenarios provide you with all-too-common experiences in the nursing profession. Think about how you'd respond, given all you've learned in this handbook. Then score yourself and see how much confidence you've gained from the communications tools in the book. Are you dauntless yet? We hope so!

Give yourself **2 points** if you know what to say when:

____ You walk into the breakroom and somebody asks you: *"Did you hear about Peggy's divorce?"*

____ The charge nurse distributes the assignment, and the first nurse that reads it sighs and rolls her eyes.

____ You walk up to the main station and two nurses are talking. One says to the other, *"What do they teach these new nurses today? She can't even do a wet to dry dressing."*

____ Coworkers constantly comment that Ginny is just plain lazy and never does her fair share, saying, *"She buddies up with the charge nurse in order to get the easiest assignments."*

2 points each for a total of 8   score = _____

Give yourself **3 points** if you know what to say when:

____ You work in the operating room. You see the surgeon hide a sponge in the sponge count to test a new nurse who is frantically re-counting.

____ A coworker walks up to you talking in a very loud voice, putting you or your work down while many others are watching and listening.

____ Your patient is three days post op. When you perform your skin assessment you notice two EKG pads on the patient's back.

___ You are swamped and see a coworker on Facebook and ask for help in turning a patient. Suddenly, the coworker stands up and says *"I'm busy and I can't."*

3 points each for a total of 12   score = _____

Give yourself **5 points** if you know what to say when:

___ You are at the main nurses' station and hear coworkers talking about a foreign-born nurse who is new to the unit. *"Don't you think that if someone comes to this country, they should be able to speak the language?"*

___ Your manager is a bully. Today she came up to you after you called out sick yesterday and said, *"How nice of you to show up for work today"* in a sarcastic tone of voice. Several people are listening. This is not the first incident.

___ Margo is avoiding you and giving you the silent treatment. You used to work well together, but something happened over a year ago when you asked her several questions about a patient. Since then the relationship has changed for the worse.

___ Your patient is scheduled for discharge to home despite the fact that she failed the home health safety evaluation. You remind the physician about the evaluation after the patient fell in the bathroom this morning. He turns briefly, looks annoyed, and simply walks away.

5 points each for a total of 20   score = _____

Total score = _____

KEY

35–40   **Expert communicator:** Dauntless, professional, and a role model for others.

25–35   **Moderate communicator:** Mastered the basic skills and positioned to become an expert with practice. Confident most of the time.

15–25   **Novice communicator:** Seek opportunities to respond, and you will gain competency and confidence.

Resources and References

Building Communication Confidence and Better Teams

In this appendix you will find important tools, video links, and bibliographic information on the literature referenced in this book.

The Dauntless App

Download the Dauntless Communication Tool app from iTunes to use as an on-the-go resource. It contains tips on how to respond to negative behaviors, a toolkit, scenarios to test your skills, and a dauntless checklist.

Team Resource: Videos for In-Service Use

The following are three short in-services designed to start the discussion on how we can all create a better work environment. You'll find links to related resources are at the end of each vignette. Allow 12 minutes for the video followed by 15–20 minutes of openly answering the questions.

Video 1: What is RN-RN Hostility?

www.youtube.com/watch?v=zrWbe7L-A1w

This 12-minute interview is followed by three discussion questions and links to handouts and other resources. The purpose of this vignette is to define and identify unprofessional behaviors and to give nurses some practical tools to take action when they witness unhealthy behaviors.

Video 2: Why Should Nurses Care About Horizontal Hostility?

www.youtube.com/watch?v=TsMaRDXJvIs

This 12-minute video connects our behaviors to our ethical obligation to keep patients safe, linking ethics to actions. Followed by three discussion questions, the video highlights why forming a team is critical to both nurses and patients.

Video 3: Communication: A Critical Tool for Creating a Healthy Work Environment

www.youtube.com/watch?v=itp962-enUI

Assertive communication is the immunization that will keep your unit healthy and your patients safe. This 12-minute video teaches the D-E-S-C communication model, explains why we don't speak up, and calls for nurses to elevate nurses from self-silencing to voice.

Additional Videos

For additional videos on culture and communication in healthcare settings, please search "Kathleen Bartholomew" at www.youtube.com.

H1 Video Simulation Tool

Spotlight-on-Healthcare is an online video simulation tool that builds communication skills for professional interactions. By practicing with Spotlight, you will build "muscle memory" and gain the confidence required to appropriately address incivility and disruptive behaviors in the workplace. Go to *http:// comassgroup.com/spotlight/* for more info.

Keep Building Your Dauntless Communication Skills

- Re-take the self-test on page 83 and compare your score with your score before you read the book. Think about the new skills you have learned.
- Cut out or copy the DESC Communication Model at the end of the book and post it where you can refer to it often.

- Cut out or copy the CR Scripting Cue Card at the end of the book and put it in your locker.
- Join our Facebook group, IamDauntless, and visit it often for dauntless communication tips.
- Visit our website, www.IamDauntless.org, for communication tips and articles. Sign-up to receive emails regarding new blog posts, read stories of how others have handled daunting communication challenges, and submit your own stories of how you have used your new found dauntless communication skills.

Bibliographic References

Allan, P. (2014). Find the perfect word for your feelings with this vocabulary wheel. Retrieved from *Lifehacker.com/find-the-perfect-word-for-your-feelings-with-this-vocab-1653513241*

Bartholomew, K. (2014). *Ending nurse-to-nurse hostility: Why nurses eat their young and each other* (2nd ed.). Danvers, MA: HCPro.

Beagan, B. L. (2003, June). Teaching social and cultural awareness to medical students: "It's all very nice to talk about in theory, but ultimately it makes no difference." *Academic Medicine, 78*(6), 605–614. Retrieved from *http://journals.lww.com/academicmedicine/Fulltext/2003/06000/ Teaching_Social_and_Cultural_Awareness_to_Medical.11.aspx*

Briles, J. (2007). Snakes at the nursing station. *American Nurse Today, 2*(8). Retrieved from *http://www.americannursetoday.com*

Brown, B. (2013). The power of vulnerability [Video file]. Retrieved from *www.ted.com/talks/brene_brown_on_vulnerability?language=en*

Budin, W. C., Brewer, C. S., Chao, Y., & Kovner, C. (2013, September).

Verbal abuse from nurse colleagues and work environment of early career registered nurses. *Journal of Nursing Scholarship, 45*(3), 308-316. http://dx.doi." org/10.1111/jnu.12033

Burgess, C., & Patton-Curry, M. (2014, April). Transforming the health care environment collaborative. *AORN Journal, 99*(4), 529-539. http://dx.doi. org/10.1016/j.aorn.2014.01.012

Ceravolo, D. J., Schwartz, D. G., Foltz-Ramos, K. M., & Castner, J. (2012). Strengthening communication to overcome lateral violence. *Journal of Nursing Management, 20*, 599-606. http://dx.doi.org/10.1111/j.1365-2834.2012.01402.x

Chu, L. (2014). Mediating toxic emotions in the workplace - the impact of abusive supervision. *Journal of Nursing Management, 22*(8), 953-963. http:// dx.doi.org/10.1111.jonm.12071

Clark, C. M. (2013). *Creating and sustaining civility in nursing education.* Indianapolis, IN: Sigma Theta Tau International Publishing.

Clippinger, J. H. (2007). *A crowd of one: The future of individual identity.* New York, NY: PublicAffairs.

Cox, D. L., & Jacobs, D. M. (2013, October 1). Measuring communication competency: The next steps in addressing disruptive behavior. *The South Carolina Nurse, 20*(4), 10. Retrieved from *http://www.scnurses.org*

Culver-Clark, R.,& Greenawald, M. (2013). Nurse-physician leadership: Insights into inter-professional collaboration. The Journal of Nursing Administration, 43(12), 653-659. http://dx.doi.org/10.1097/NNA.0000000000000007

D'Ambra, A. M., & Andrews, D. R. (2014). Incivility, retention and new graduate nurses: An integrated review of the literature. *Journal of Nursing Management, 22*(6), 735-742. http://dx.doi.org/10.1111/jonm.12060

Finkelman, A., & Kenner, C. (2012). *Teaching IOM: Implications of the Institute of Medicine reports for nursing education* (3rd ed.). Silver Springs, MD: American Nurses Association.

Fousey. (2013, December 1). *The Bullying Experiment* [Video file]. Retrieved from *ww.youtube.com: Fouseytube The Bullying Experiment.*

Freire, P. (1990). *Pedagogy of the oppressed* (4th ed.). New York, NY: Continuum International.

Griffin, M., & Clark, C. M. (2014, November 22). Revisiting cognitive rehearsal as an intervention against incivility and lateral violence in nursing: 10 years later. *The Journal of Continuing Education in Nursing, 45*(12), 535-542. http:// dx.doi.org/10.3928/00220124-20141122-02

Haidt, J. (2012). *The Righteous Mind: Why Good People Are Divided by Politics and Religion.* New York: Pantheon Books.

Hannah, C. F. (2006). Scapegoating and the unpopular nurse. *Nurse Education Today, 11*(4). http://dx.doi.org/10.1016/j.nedt.2006.11.004

King-Jones, M. (2011). Horizontal violence and the socialization of new nurses. *Creative Nursing, 17*(2), 80–86. http://dx.doi.org/10.1891/1078-4535.17.2.80

Kritek, P. B. (2002). *Negotiating at an uneven table: Developing moral courage in resolving our conflicts* (2nd ed.). San Francisco, CA: Jossey-Bass.

Lachman, V. D. (2015). Ethical issues in the disruptive behaviors of incivility, bullying, and horizontal/lateral violence. *Journal of Urologic Nurses and Associates, 35*(1), 39–42. Retrieved from *http://www.medscape.com/viewarticle/841143*

Longhurst, C. (2016). Gossip can help to stop poor care, claims study. *Nursing Standard, 31*(8). Http:dx.doi.org/10.7748/ns.31.8.10.s8

Maxfield, D., Grenny, J., Lavandero, R., & Groah, L. (2010). The silent treatment: Why safety tools and checklists aren't enough to save lives. Retrieved from http://www.aacn.org/wd/hwe/docs/the-silent-treatment.pdf

Mitchell, A., Ahmed, A., & Szabo, C. (2014, February 13). Workplace violence among nurses, why are we still discussing this? Literature review. *Journal of Nursing Education and Practice, 4*(4), 147–150. http://dx.doi.org/10.5430/jnep.v4n4p147

Norgaard, B., Ammentorp, J., Kyvik, K. O., & Kofoed, P. (2012). Communication skills training increases self-efficacy of health care professionals. *Journal of Continuing Education in the Health Professions, 32*(2), 90–97. *https://www.researchgate.net/journal/1554-558X_Journal_of_Continuing_Education_in_the_Health_Professions*

Patterson, K., Grenny, J., McMillan, R., & Switzler, A. (2012). *Crucial conversations: Tools for talking when stakes are high* (2nd ed.). New York, NY: McGraw Hill.

Porath, C. & Erez, A. (2007). Does rudeness really matter? The effects of rudeness on task performance and helpfulness. *Academy of Management Journal 50(5): 1181-1197.*

Roberts, S. J., & Clarke, P. N. (2015). Lateral violence in nursing: A review of the past three decades. *Nursing Science Quarterly, 28*(1), 36–41. http://dx.doi. org/10.1177/0894318414558614

Robins, A. K. (2015). *A history of violence: Communicating to stop horizontal hostility*. Unpublished manuscript, Department of Nursing and Health Sciences, Grand Canyon University, Phoenix, AZ.

Scrubs. (2013). A list of rules for nurses from 1887. Retrieved from *http://scrubsmag.com/a-list-of-rules-for-nurses-from-1887/*

Stagg, S. J., Sheridan, D., Jones, R. A., & Speroni, K. G. (2011). Evaluation of a workplace bullying cognitive rehearsal program in a hospital setting. *The Journal of Continuing Education in Nursing, 42*(9), 395–401. http://dx.doi.org/10.3928/00220124-20110823-22

Swift, T. (2010). Mean. On Speak Now [CD]. Retrieved from *https://www.youtube.com/watch?v=jYaleIlhpDE*

Symer, L. S., Hynes, G., & Hall, K. L. (2012, September 1). Strategies for teaching social and emotional intelligence in business communication. Business Communication Quarterly, 75(3), 309–317. http://dx.doi.org/10.1177/1080569912450312

Thompson, D., & Marstiller, J. (2010). Conflict resolution. Retrieved from *http://www.ahrq.gov/professionals/education/curriculum-tools/cusptoolkit/ toolkit/contentcalls/conflict_resolution-slides/conflictresslides.html*

Walrafen, N., Brewer, M. K., & Mulvenon, C. (2012). Sadly caught up in the moment: An exploration of horizontal violence. *Nursing Economic$, 30*(1), 6–12, 49.

Weick, Karl E. & Sutcliffe, Kathleen M. (2015). *Managing the Unexpected* (3rd Ed.) Hoboken, NJ: John Wiley & Sons, Inc.

Wing, T., Regan, S., & Spence-Laschinger, H. K. (2015, July). The influence of empowerment and incivility on the mental health of new graduate nurses. *Journal of Nursing Management, 23*(5), 632–643. http://dx.doi.org/10.1111/jonm.12190

Cut out this page and post it somewhere (such as your locker) as a reminder of how to handle communication conflicts in a professional manner.

Courageous Communicator	
The DESC Communication Model	
Describe	**D**escribe the situation: *"When... happened..."*
Explore	**E**xplore or express your thoughts, feelings or concerns *"I felt..."* Phrase your response (when appropriate) to give the benefit of the doubt: *"Was it your intent to...?"*
— Pause —	
State	**S**tate what you want to do differently next time: *"In the future, would you...?"*
Consequence	**C**onsequence: State the positive consequence when they do as you ask.

Cut out the following cue card and keep it somewhere (such as in your badge holder or locker) you can quickly refer to it.

SCRIPTING CUE CARD

Possible Pre-Rehearsed Responses:

1. **Non-verbal innuendo** (raising of eyebrows, face-making)
   - *I sense (I see from your facial expression) that there may be something you wanted to address with me. It's okay to speak with me directly.*
2. **Verbal affront** (covert/overt, snide remarks, lack of openness, abrupt responses)
   - *The individuals that I learn the most from are clearer in their directions and feedback. Is there some way we can structure this type of learning situation?*
   - *That may be information I don't need to know/hear. What would help me is...*
3. **Undermining** (turning away, not available)
   - *When an event happens that is contrary to my understanding, it leaves me with questions. Help me understand how this situation happened.*
4. **Withholding information** (practice or patient)
   - *It is my understanding that there is (was) more information available regarding this situation, and I believe that if I had known that, it would (will) affect how I handle what I learn or need to know.*
5. **Sabotage** (deliberate setting up of a situation)
   - *There is more to this situation than meets the eye. Could "you and I" (whatever/whomever) meet in private and explore what happened?*

6. **Infighting** (bickering with peers—open contentious discussion is unprofessional and should be avoided)
   - *This is not the time or place—please stop.* (physically move to a neutral spot)
   - *I'm moving to another location.*
7. **Scapegoating** (attributing all that goes wrong to one individual—rarely is one individual, incident, situation the cause for all that goes wrong. Scapegoating is an easy route to travel, but rarely solves problems.)
   - *I don't think that is the right connection.*
8. **Backstabbing** (complaining to others about an individual but not speaking to that individual—like scapegoating, is maladaptive and nonproductive.)
   - *It's not right to talk about someone when they are not here. Have you spoken to her directly about your concerns?*
9. **Failure to respect**
   - *It bothers me to talk about that without their permission.*
   - *I only overheard that. It shouldn't be repeated.*
10. **Broken confidences**
    - *Wasn't that said in confidence?*
    - *That sounds like information that should remain confidential.*
    - *He/she asked me to keep that confidential.*

Adapted from Effective Communication (Glod, 1998) for Cognitive Rehearsal by M. Griffin, RN CS, PhD (2003)

What Nursing Leaders Are Saying About *The Dauntless Nurse:*

Workplace bullying in healthcare organizations can have devastating and far-reaching effects, and if left unaddressed, can potentially result in patient injury or death. The stakes are far too high for nurses to remain silent. This wonderfully written book authored by three experts on nurse bullying is jam-packed with evidence-based, practical, ready-to-use tips and tools to Ctrl+Alt+Delete these damaging behaviors. The authors provide readers with a wide range of communication strategies to help nurses boost their moral courage, exercise their voice, and become dauntless advocates for patient safety. This inspiring book is replete with valuable tools to help nurses reframe their inner dialogue to create a new story where courageous individuals and high performing teams provide a durable safety net for patient care. This book is a must-read for every healthcare professional wishing to build their confidence and expand their ability to address conflicted situations.

Cynthia Clark, PhD, RN, ANEF, FAAN
Strategic Nursing Advisor & Consultant, ATI Nursing Education
Professor Emeritus, Boise State University
Author of *Creating and Sustaining Civility in Nursing Education*

The Dauntless Nurse: Communication Confidence Builder published by Martha E. Griffin, Kathleen Bartholomew and Arna Robins is a wonderfully written practical guide for practicing nurses in all work environments where communication confidence is needed for one's own professional development and the ultimate safety of patients. Speaking up and not silencing one's voice is key in the development of the ability "to care to confront" hard issues. Cognitive rehearsal and subsequent self and patient advocacy techniques is a fundamental skill to which all nurses in every workplace need to aspire. This book gives many examples and helpful hints to advance the ability of nurses to be courageous, tenacious, and honest in direct communication when it is easier to do just the opposite.

Rosanna DeMarco, PhD, RN, PHCNS-BC, APHN-FAAN

The Dauntless Nurse is an excellent book for all nurses, especially new graduates and students, who find themselves in a work situation where bullying and lateral violence are predominant. This reading gives concrete and helpful ways to learn how to communicate with the nurses who bully other nurses. You can learn how to change your behavior so that you can make a positive and creative response in these difficult situations. Changing your own behavior can change the negative cycle of interactions between nurses and make your life and the care for your patients so much better. I highly endorse it!!

Susan J Roberts, DNSc, ANP, FAAN
Professor of Nursing
Northeastern University School of Nursing